The Russian Affair

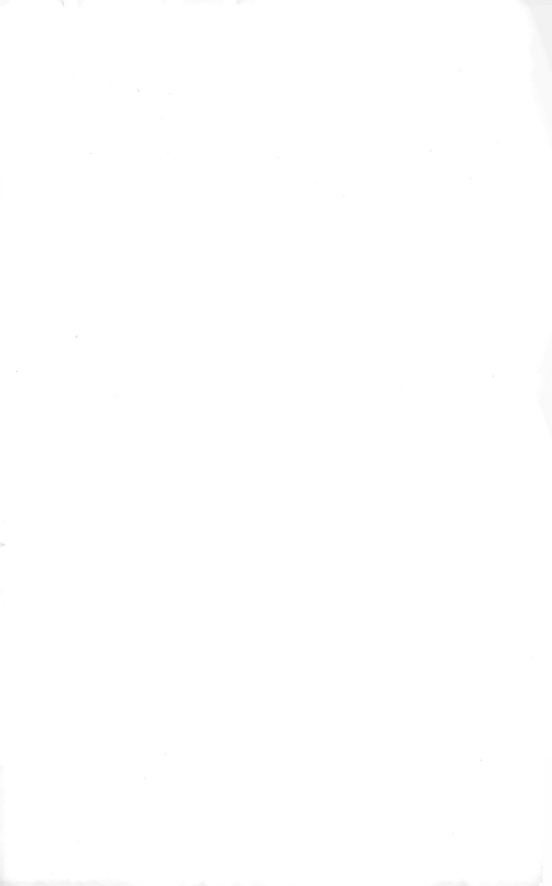

The Russian Affair

THE TRUE STORY OF THE COUPLE WHO DISCOVERED THE GREATEST SPORTING SCANDAL

David Walsh

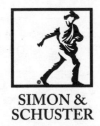

SIMON &
SCHUSTER

London · New York · Sydney · Toronto · New Delhi

First published in Great Britain by Simon & Schuster UK Ltd, 2020

1 3 5 7 9 10 8 6 4 2

Simon & Schuster UK Ltd
1st Floor
222 Gray's Inn Road
London WC1X 8HB

www.simonandschuster.co.uk
www.simonandschuster.com.au
www.simonandschuster.co.in

Simon & Schuster Australia, Sydney
Simon & Schuster India, New Delhi

A CIP catalogue record for this book
is available from the British Library

Hardback ISBN: 978-1-4711-5815-5
Trade Paperback ISBN: 978-1-4711-5816-2
eBook ISBN: 978-1-4711-5817-9

Typeset in Bembo by M Rules
Printed and bound by CPI Group (UK) Ltd, Croydon, CR0 4YY

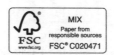

MIX
Paper from
responsible sources
FSC® C020471
FSC
www.fsc.org

Foreword

On Wednesday 7 January 2015, I travelled to Berlin to meet Vitaly and Yuliya Stepanov for the first time. The investigative journalist Hajo Seppelt had been the go-between for our meeting. When the four of us gathered at a small cafe, Vitaly and I began a conversation that has rumbled on for five years. One question has dominated all others: why? Why would a lowly doping control officer working for Rusada, the Russian Anti-Doping Agency, turn spy? Especially as his wife was an elite athlete and part of the system?

Seppelt had made a fine documentary, *Top Secret Doping – How Russia Makes Its Winners*, for German state television, which had broadcast it five weeks earlier. In the opening credits Vitaly and Yuliya are seen strolling through a Moscow park with their one-year-old son, Robert. They are lit by sunshine, the trees are leafy green, life seems idyllic. Then Vitaly and Seppelt are shown sitting at a table in an empty restaurant. Vitaly explains what motivated him to join Russia's anti-doping agency.

'I wanted to fight doping and I wanted to make sports cleaner. More honest. Better. I truly believed that I came to work for an anti-doping organisation who will fight doping. And I was not married back then, I was single. I was ready to work twenty-four hours a day.'

Something about this quiet, matter-of-fact expression of idealism struck me as odd. What was it about this guy? Doping was a well-funded, state-supported service for Russia's athletes, viewed as a means of enhancing the global reputation of Mother Russia. The conspiracy involved every sports organisation in the country, every government agency and, of course, the Ministry of Sport. How could one small cog – in the midst of so many interlocking and free-moving wheels – think he could make any difference?

If you think that you are too small to make a difference, ask a mosquito.

After joining Rusada, Vitaly remained single for not much more than a year. His relationship with Yuliya would be complex. He was a dreamer. She was a tough pragmatist. They married each other anyway. The anti-doping zealot and the committed doper. How could that work? Vitaly's devotion to anti-doping was intriguing, but his marriage was perplexing.

Now here they were in Berlin. At the end of one journey, and at the beginning of another. The only certainty was that the second part of their lives would be nothing like the first. In the blink of an eye, their home in Moscow had become their past. They'd had to get out before Seppelt told the world that Russia was the biggest cheat in sport. Six weeks into their exile, they knew they would not be able to go back.

'Financially, what's your situation?'

'Not good.'

'How will you survive?'

'If we can find a country that will take us, we will work.'

'You could earn some money if you wrote a book.'

'Would you help us to do that?'

And so began *The Russian Affair*.

PART ONE

You will not grasp her with your mind
Or cover with a common label,
For Russia is one of a kind—
Believe in her, if you are able.

Fyodor Tyutchev,
Russian poet, 1803–73

Prologue

Monday afternoon 3 August 2009, offices of Rusada, the Russian anti-doping agency, close to Moscow's Kiyevsky station. Conversation between Vitaly Stepanov and Director Vyacheslav Sinev

'Director Sinev, do you have a moment?'

'Vitaly, for you I have several moments.'

'I was out on a date last night.'

'A date! On a Sunday? Well, that is allowed, Vitaly! Life isn't about Outreach alone. Will this be happening again?'

'Well, I need to talk to you about something that happened.'

'On your date?'

'Yes.'

'Of course. Just not too much information so soon after my lunch, please, Vitaly.'

'She was an athlete.'

'But this morning she has retired, right?'

'No. She is still an athlete, but she told me certain things.'

'Oh, okay.'

'I thought you might need to hear them.'

'Do proceed, Vitaly, but bear in mind that myself and Mrs Sinev are already people of the world. We aren't easily shocked.'

'She told me that she is doping.'

'I see. That was refreshingly frank.'

'And that everybody she knows is also doping. She said that the coaches don't regard doping as cheating. She said they think that Rusada is just there to help them.'

'Hmm. Well, she sounds like an interesting girl.'

'I just thought I should tell you.'

'Yes. Of course, Vitaly. Of course. Thank you for the information. Quite a first date. My advice to you is don't get too involved with the girl. Two words, my friend: be careful.'

Chapter 1

Several days earlier

Vitaly smiled. Things were going well.

At his desk in Moscow he sorted through the data from the Outreach trip in Cheboksary. Athletes had filled out questionnaires and Vitaly had inputted their responses and contact details into his database. The answers weren't convincing, and it had taken the lure of free gifts to get athletes to engage, but what Vitaly had now was better than nothing.

How odd, he thought as he came across three forms from the same runner. He soon realised this was not an outlier in terms of enthusiasm; a different gift had been claimed each time. *Very odd.* He'd given her one himself but the other two had been handed over by his colleague Alexey. *What the . . . ? Aha, it was that blonde 800 metres runner, the blue-eyed one with the techno-buns hairstyle. Cheeky! And Alexey, you dog, what were you thinking?* Vitaly grinned. She looked like a bit of an operator, this young woman.

It was true that Yuliya Rusanova had turned up at the Outreach not to learn anything about doping but to get as many gifts as she could. If she remembered Vitaly Stepanov at all, it was because her friend Oksana Khaleeva had been trying to match her up with him.

'My friend here, she's not attached. She's a good girl.'

5

'No, no, no,' said the good girl, conveying the impression that her dance card was full, thank you.

Pity, Vitaly had thought to himself at the time. But maybe there was no need to abandon all hope after all. He called up the social network site Odnoklassniki and sent Ms Techno-Buns some photos taken at the stand, making a little joke out of her three-gift heist.

Yuliya Rusanova from Kursk. There was something about her.

She responded with a bare-bones 'thank you', but it came back quickly enough to encourage him. Or rather not to discourage him, so he sent another message.

The conversation was flirty, at least when he was typing. If Kursk hadn't been more than 300 miles away he would have asked her straight out for a date. She threw him a crumb, though, letting it slip that she was catching a flight to a competition on the following Monday morning and that she would be spending the night before with a relative who lived near the airport at Domodedovo.

'Maybe I could give you a call,' Vitaly said.

'Maybe,' she replied, as if all things were possible but of equal insignificance to her.

The following weekend he was again on Outreach duty, this time at the World Junior Canoe and Kayak Championships in Krylatskoye, Moscow. Vitaly loved his work but he was distracted. By Sunday afternoon he was keen to wrap up and see if he could catch up with this runner from Kursk. He called her mid-afternoon, suggesting they meet up at around seven o'clock. She agreed in a way that again made her indifference plain. He settled for that.

First, though, Vitaly would have to drive his colleague Oleg Samsonov back to his apartment in the centre of Moscow. That meant driving all the way into the city before coming back out. Doable.

Around five o'clock she called him: 'Look, I'm sorry but I am not feeling well, and I've got an early flight tomorrow. Can we just cancel?'

'Well, I'm actually already on the way there.'

'Oh, okay. Well, if you are already driving then you may as well come.'

She sounded disappointed. Not a good start, having a date disappointed that the date was actually going to happen. But she asked him to pick her up at the apartment building next to the one she was staying in.

When he arrived she slipped confidently into the passenger seat.

'What's this?' she said, glancing over her left shoulder at the baby seat he used when driving his toddler cousin, Stepan, around Moscow.

'I have two kids,' he said, 'but don't worry, I didn't tell my wife I was coming.'

Her smile was as cold and thin as a razor blade. If she detected the joke in his patter, she wasn't acknowledging it. This might be hard work. He'd come bearing gifts, though: all five items in the Outreach range. Her expression softened a little.

They drove in search of a takeaway and then talked in the car while they ate. He wondered if he wasn't reaching for something beyond his grasp. She was training to be an Olympic and World champion, whereas his job was collecting the urine of would-be champions. Yet one thing made him different from most young Russian men: he'd been somewhere. *Play that card, Vitaly.* And so he told her about New York.

'What's the one thing everyone now remembers about New York?' he asked her. 'Yes, that thing!' He had been there when that had happened. It was a long story, not one to cut short.

He'd had this apartment there. He could see the river. One Monday night he stayed up too late, just watching *Forrest Gump* on his widescreen TV. He loved that movie. That feather. How it floated down so soft and random through the opening credits and dropped between Tom Hanks' feet as he sat on his bench at the bus stop. How he took it and placed it tenderly between the leaves of his picture book in his small, tidy case. Vitaly had got that. Totally.

'It's not some story about a simpleton who eats chocolates,' he told her. 'If that's what you've heard, it's not. It's about running. A lot of it is about running.'

When the alarm had buzzed the next morning, Vitaly hit snooze. When he next woke up he realised he had overslept. He was supposed to have been in Citibank an hour ago, talking to a man about why the bank might loan Vitaly some money. The apartment was too expensive really. He knew that. One wall of his bedroom was just glass. Imagine. That morning he just lay back and enjoyed it. Citibank would wait.

'In New York, you see, it's different. The customer is the king over there.'

Vitaly was a day trader. Not so much a trade as a hobby. He'd read some parts of some books on day trading. Introductions, chapters one and two. He'd had some early luck. It wasn't coal mining, it wasn't rocket science, it wasn't full-time. He did a lot of running and a little day trading. A good work–life balance, he thought.

As he got out of bed, Vitaly heard the whickering blades of a helicopter outside his window. He saw the machine float slowly down towards the strip of green parkland that separated his building from the Hudson River. There was always something going on in New York City. Down below, when he looked, there were people gathering on the grass. He played pick-up games of soccer down there on bright evenings, but he'd never seen a helicopter land there. Nor so many people.

In the lounge he switched on the big television. It had taken four men to manoeuvre that giant screen into place. Excessive, but really it was the mother of all televisions. The picture was as vivid as the view out the window. He'd paid extra to be on this side of the building, on River Terrace, with the view of the Hudson. On the other side of the building the apartments were cheaper and they looked out toward the World Trade Center. On his TV screen now that's what they were showing. Those sharp lines of the twin towers cleaved by the blue rectangle of September sky.

It took a moment for him to register what he was watching. A dense plume of smoke was rising from the north tower as if billowing from the ear of a very tall man. CNBC said that a plane had crashed into the tower. The building had swallowed the plane like some kind of bug. It was the tower in which Vitaly had been scheduled to have his Citibank meeting this morning. He sat down and stared, and as he watched the other tower was hit.

How strangely the mind works. A large plane had just flown into the building down the street. He'd barely heard a sound. That's how top-end the finish on the apartment was. Then he began to shake. Two planes had smashed into a building down the street.

He called home. Elena, his mother, answered. Vitaly explained what had happened and reassured her: 'All good? Isn't it always, Mum? You know me. Talk later.' He called friends who he thought might worry, and said the same words.

He watched TV until the woman from CNBC said, 'Oh my god,' and one tower just folded in on itself. Then the TV got shut down. The power in the building went off. Vitaly shook some more. He stuffed things into a backpack. The elevator ran off a separate generator in the building and it was still functioning. When the doors opened there was a man already in the lift. He and Vitaly were the last people to leave the building. The man had no idea where his wife and children were. In the lobby they told each other to be safe and then they headed in different directions.

The outside world was nothing but smoke and dust. Vitaly moved northwards until he realised that if they were taking down landmarks perhaps it was best not to be near the Empire State Building, so he turned west, towards the Hudson. At Pier 25, like a spirit leaving his body, his fear disappeared. *If something explodes*, he thought, *I will swim*. People stood and waited. Some wept. Vitaly stood and waited with them. In time a boat appeared. The captain wanted to ferry injured people to Jersey City but there were no injured at Pier 25 yet. Just these waiting, weeping people. The captain filled his boat anyway.

At Jersey City Vitaly found a church. The priest greeted him like a friend, took him to the parish house and gestured towards the phone. Vitaly rang Elena again, telling her it was all good, all okay, and promised to call again in forty-eight hours.

The injured began to arrive at the church, and Vitaly joined an improvised help crew. The following days would melt into one long day. Bandages. Splints. Wounds. Crying. Tears. Sounds. Smells.

A family took Vitaly and other strangers into their apartment. They were all one now. The building was old and squat, no more than three storeys tall but in the evenings from the roof you could watch lower Manhattan in its ruin. People did so many small good things in Jersey City that week. Every evening Vitaly looked across the river and knew that there were people over there doing bigger, braver things.

He wondered what would have happened had he died. His grieving parents having to splice together the loose ends of their son's strange life. Mourning his death and the $200,000 Vitaly had cost them since he was sent to America as a fifteen-year-old to learn English. Death would have revealed him as weak, irresponsible, less than the son they'd hoped he'd be. He thought how much better it would be to live the life of an honest and humble man. It was then that he knew it was time to turn his eyes towards the place he was born.

When he'd finished talking, his New York story had taken longer than he'd planned and he wasn't too sure why he'd started. Was he talking too much?

He asked Yuliya about her earliest memory.

Her stories were different. First, a story she knew from Nadia, her grandmother. Yuliya was two years old. They lived in a green wooden house on a nature reserve 18 kilometres from Kursk. There was her sister, Katia, who was three years older and her parents, Igor and Lyubov. They lived there because Igor loved nature and worked on the reserve. He was good with animals. Once, he and Lyubov found two abandoned baby wolves, brought them home and raised them as pets. They behaved not much differently from dogs. Another time Igor brought home an injured wild pig, nursed it back to health and then kept it in the enclosed yard around their house. Though domesticated, the pig snapped at the dogs and cats. Igor named the pig Lyubov because he said the pig annoyed him in the same way his wife did. It became a family joke.

Sometimes bad weather came and left them without electricity. One such evening, when Igor and Lyubov were out, Nadia was looking after the girls and at dusk the wolves, attracted as usual by the smell of the domestic animals, began to howl. Katia was Yuliya's guardian angel. When Yuliya asked about the noises outside, Katia replied, 'Wolves, sister. They are wolves.' They came at this time most evenings, but in the dark it was worse.

'Be quiet and the wolves will never know we are here,' Katia would tell her.

Yuliya couldn't have spoken even if she'd wanted to. And they would sit in silence on the wooden stairs, holding each other, frozen in the sheer blackness.

Darkness, Vitaly thought. He'd seen some bad things; she'd lived them. He'd been to New York; she'd had wolves as pets.

They spoke about their current situations.

Was she attached? 'No, not really.'

Him? 'Same.'

'Good.'

'Yeah, good.'

She asked him what exactly he did at Rusada. He said he collected urine samples and worked in the area of education. Rusada was trying to raise awareness about the problem of doping. He dropped in some of his own thoughts about how he saw the fight going.

He sensed already she was someone that he might never fully know. She was like a closed city. Areas of her brain seemed folded away in places nobody could be granted permission to travel in. There was also the possibility that she just found him boring. Her distracted expression warned him that maybe the clock was running down on his audition. Thank you for a lovely evening. Next?

His work background wasn't great material. He worried that she was about to ask what he thought he would do when he grew up. Or if his job came with a little uniform.

She didn't. She simply said, 'You really should just stop being an idiot.'

She didn't think he was right. About anything. She wondered if he could really be so clueless. Her coach was for ever making arrangements with Rusada. If there was a problem, who was he going to call? Rusada. A little shaken, Vitaly clung to the cliff edge.

'So, if your coach is "helping you",' he said, 'does that mean you are doping as well?'

'Look, everybody is using doping.'

'Really?'

'And Rusada knows everybody dopes. They help us. I am using doping, everyone is using doping. Rusada is there to help us be dirty.'

He started the car and pulled away, just so he could keep his eyes on the road while she spoke.

'It's not like I'm breaking the rules,' she said. 'These *are* the rules.'

Now he was really listening. She saw no danger in telling him what it was like to be a Russian athlete. He couldn't help admiring her up-front 'take it or leave it' delivery.

'To be a top athlete, this is what it takes,' she said. 'End of lesson.'

Her phone rang, giving him a moment to think. There were two thoughts.

What she was telling him was certainly the basis for an investigation. He should ask more questions, make some mental notes, get more understanding of the world he was dealing with. This could be the start of a major professional coup. He could break an entire doping ring because he had driven here to see this girl. Alternatively, when she got off the phone he could just ask her for a second date. She was something else, this Yuliya Rusanova.

She was speaking with another athlete from Kursk, a girl called Kristina Khaleeva. An up-and-comer in the middle distances and Oksana's older sister. Vitaly knew the name. Khaleeva was helping Yuliya to get a contract to run for the police in the Korolev district of Moscow suburbs. The state had various ways of rewarding its athletes, one of which was for an athlete to compete for a police division or an army sector. The athlete turned up a couple of times a year, ran then posed for pictures. There was a monthly income and various protections, including a pension.

Yuliya was agitated. Khaleeva had been talking her up to a contact in the police but she had said too much.

'Why the fuck did you tell him about my father?' Yuliya was saying.

A pause as Khaleeva defended herself.

This is interesting, thought Vitaly. *What has your father done that you don't want the Korolev police to know about?* Vitaly hadn't known that many women, but this one was definitely the most intriguing.

Yuliya Rusanova flapped her hand at Vitaly.

'Stop the car.'

He obeyed instantly. *Now I'm just her driver.*

'This is a real problem for me, Kristina,' she was saying. 'It's no good being sorry, Kristina.'

She stepped out of the car and continued the conversation outside. Vitaly leaned his head back on the headrest, closed his eyes and let out a long, slow breath. Wow.

Presently she returned to the car. Still agitated. Her friend had screwed up, she said. Anyway, she was taking an early flight from Domodedovo airport the next morning.

'Time to go,' she said.

'I'd like to see you again,' he said.

She sighed.

Would she mind if he came back in the morning and drove her to the airport?

Now she frowned. Her first thought: *This guy is like a puppy looking for affection.* Her second thought: *I won't have to pay for a cab.*

'If you want to,' she said.

When he'd asked the question, he'd intended to drive back to his apartment in Moscow, getting up super early and returning. Now he had a change of heart. He thought of the journey back, how long it would take, then the early-morning start.

'I'll sleep in the car near the apartment building. In the morning, when you are ready, just come outside.'

'You don't have to try so hard to show me you are a good guy, you know. Stay here all night? Are you completely crazy?'

'Maybe,' he said.

~

Yuliya departed Domodedovo early that Monday morning. Her manager, Sergey Nochevniy, had made the travel arrangements. Three flights and fifteen hours just to get to Castres in the south of France. Bloody Sergey. He could complicate a two-car funeral.

Travelling all day, she thought from time to time about the guy from the night before and graded the date. He'd waited dutifully outside all night to taxi her. That was a new one. Otherwise? She wouldn't have said he was boring but he was no roller-coaster ride. And seriously, she actually did know how sport worked in Russia. She didn't need the lesson, thank you all the same. Maybe it was just the usual first-date wonder-of-me bullshit but there was really no need for it. She'd held back, waiting for him to realise that he was preaching to the wrong congregation, but he seemed to be deadly serious. He wasn't a pen-pushing underling happy to have a state job at Rusada. He really wanted to run about, fighting doping like some gallant knight on his white charger. You meet all sorts.

It was late and dark when she got to her sleepy French hotel but it was sunny when she woke the next morning. She really needed to get rid of bloody Sergey.

Chapter 2

Spring/early summer 2008

Olga, who had been Vitaly's previous girlfriend, left him not long after he got the job at Rusada.

'Vitaly,' she said, 'they haven't paid you any money yet.'

This was true. He lived on tinned food.

'Vitaly,' she said, 'you have these ideals but no income. I don't need a man who works for nothing. You can't spend ideals.'

It was true that many of the people who had started work with Vitaly a couple of months ago had quit. They felt the same way as Olga did about the 'no income' thing.

'Not committed,' Director Sinev said of the vanished people. 'This is a job for people who care about sport. There's a silver lining, though, Vitaly. You have been with Rusada for a month and already you are the senior employee!'

Vyacheslav Sinev was the new sheriff in a town that wasn't sure it needed a sheriff. Rusada had been established to organise the fight against doping in Russia. This was how Vitaly saw it. It was a good and just cause requiring a good and just plan. But there was no plan. No plan, no resources, no wages and – from what Vitaly could see – not much enthusiasm for the battle ahead. Director Sinev swore that the people at the Federal Agency for Physical Education and Sports (known as Rossport) were cutting through reams of red tape, even as he spoke. Money would flow. Rusada would grow. Every little thing was going to be all right.

'Relax, Vitaly,' Director Sinev said. 'Relax. This is Russia. Things take time.'

Fine, but Olga just wasn't the patient type.

Vitaly chose to believe in Director Sinev. Every country needed its anti-doping agency. Yes, it was true that Rusada didn't have its own offices. The staff squatted in three rooms at the end of a long corridor in a shabby old building belonging to Rossport on Kazakova Street. True too that staff just came and went at Rusada. Nobody knew what they were doing or how long they might do it for. They passed their days making vague plans and worrying about the early-evening traffic. Most were gone within weeks.

Vitaly made himself useful when he could and turned up when he should and only left when there was nothing to keep him at work or when he needed to avoid the worst of Moscow's traffic. Those wageless weeks brought a sort of freedom but also a sense of purpose. Vitaly held on to the ideal. Why else would they be there but for clean sport?

Previously his life was notable for all the things that he started but didn't finish. Mainly courses and careers. That was the old Vitaly, though. He'd seen *The Untouchables* and he liked the way that Eliot Ness cleaned up Chicago. A lot of Chicago's bad guys had sniggered at Ness in the early days, but it had all worked out in the end. Vitaly would hang in there, but there were things afoot that even Eliot Ness didn't have to deal with.

Early one evening in Rusada's office, he was thinking about packing it in for the day. Things had improved, wages had arrived and, although Vitaly didn't mind staying late, this was one day when he wished he'd gone home early. He was staring at Tatyana Lysenko, world-record holder for the hammer throw. Director Sinev had mentioned her, almost lasciviously, and Vitaly could now see what all that was about.

Lysenko was from Rostov-on-Don and had been in the news recently.[1] She and another Rostov thrower, Yekaterina Khoroshikh, had been discovered by a local coach called Nikolai Beloborodov.[2] From nowhere Lysenko came to throw a world-record 77.06 metres in July 2005.[3] She had not just overtaken the old mark but pinned it up against the ropes and pummelled it. That evening in Moscow she'd thrown almost a metre further than any woman in history.

Two days later, in Germany, Khoroshikh won the European Under-23 title, throwing a championship-record 71.51 metres. Her throw landed almost two metres further than that of the runner-up and was more than three metres better than her personal best.

Beloborodov merely had to keep his two women out of trouble until the Beijing Games, but that proved too much. Now, for some reason, the trouble had come to Vitaly's door.

At Lysenko's shoulder stood Dr Grigory Rodchenkov. In the anti-doping world Rodchenkov was perhaps the single most important man in Russia. Tall and thin with tinted teardrop glasses and a droopy moustache which lent him a gloomy air, Rodchenkov was director of the Moscow anti-doping laboratory. He had been a decent athlete and it was known that he himself had experimented with performance-enhancing drugs. Now he was more widely recognised as a world authority on such drugs and their detection. He'd been published and peer-reviewed. He'd travelled regularly to international conferences and spoken about anti-doping. People understood that he knew his subject. Yet this wasn't the sanitised world of a world anti-doping conference but a private encounter among Russians. Only Russians.

Rodchenkov wanted Vitaly to accompany Lysenko to the bathroom and watch as she delivered a urine sample. Rodchenkov and Vitaly both knew this was against the rules.

Ms Lysenko had to be accompanied by a person of her own gender. Rodchenkov conceded the point and said that he would be happy if Vitaly preferred to limit his supervisory duties to the completion of the doping form and the division of the sample into the A and B bottles. There was no need for him to watch Ms Lysenko actually express the sample.

'But if nobody monitors then it will not be a valid sample,' said Vitaly.

'Well then, watch if you need to.'

'No, I don't need to and you know that what you are suggesting is not proper or ethical.'

Vitaly shouldn't have been surprised. The early days at Rusada coincided with an especially weird and interesting time in Russian sport.[4] Amid all the recent scandals, a doping story about two hammer throwers from Rostov-on-Don wasn't anybody's idea of big news. But whatever kind of story Lysenko was, Vitaly just didn't need to be in it.

Lysenko and Khoroshikh had come up positive following an out-of-competition doping control in Moscow a year earlier. The test was administered by the World Anti-Doping Agency (WADA) and the samples sent to a laboratory in Lausanne. Nikolai Beloborodov was furious. His throwers declined to have their B samples analysed, claiming a legal supplement sold to them by the head coach of the national team, Mr Valery Kulichenko, had contained the banned substance. It was a familiar story made more interesting by Beloborodov fingering a coach who was part of the establishment.

Kulichenko was a throwback. The Russia he knew was part of the Soviet Union, where difficulties such as these just vanished. How was WADA allowed to come to Moscow and test? In the old days a coach successfully applying 'special methods' was rewarded with a nice car, a decent apartment, perhaps a dacha in the countryside. In the new world, old practices evolved. Now a coach was free to keep whatever he could earn by his own enterprise.

Beloborodov's accusations were passed upwards to the director of the Centre of Sport Training right here in the Rossport building. Surprisingly Kulichenko was suspended until the investigation was complete. He was apoplectic. Who were these hammer throwers anyway? Where was the loyalty, the gratitude, the respect? He hit back.

'I am not the rascal . . . most interesting is the fact that nobody has proved yet that the substance found in the samples of the girls is doping . . . The director of the Russian Anti-Doping Laboratory Grigory Rodchenkov gave the conclusion that it is not doping . . . nothing is clear yet, and mud has been flung in my direction . . . I had a micro heart attack in Tula. For the moment I am in bed again, and what do I learn?'

Rodchenkov stood in front of Vitaly now and said, 'I have to check Ms Lysenko's sample quickly because it might be possible that she will go to Beijing. Please do as I ask.'

The Olympics were weeks away. Tatyana Lysenko was a banned athlete. Vitaly couldn't see how this might happen or why he had to be involved. Vitaly himself had translated the protocols of the WADA code on testing.

The athlete will be asked to provide a urine sample of at least 90ml under direct observation of a DCO [Doping Control Officer] or witnessing chaperone of the same gender. In order for the DCO or chaperone to have a clear view of the sample being provided, the athlete will be asked to pull their shirt up to mid-torso and trousers down to mid-thigh. As soon as the athlete has finished providing the sample, the DCO or chaperone will instruct the athlete to immediately secure the vessel with the lid.

'A clear view.' This was awkward.

In January 2008 Rodchenkov had been dragged into the Lysenko affair. The athlete had said in November that she handed over the contentious supplement to Rodchenkov for testing. In person. Rodchenkov said this never happened. Lysenko was baffled, but Rodchenkov was adamant. Lysenko said that the supplement must have somehow disappeared. No, said Rodchenkov, he had never seen it. Rodchenkov said that when the story broke in the summer of 2007, he had – out of professional interest – attempted to buy some of the supplement as he wished to test it privately. He had been told it was no longer available. Having encountered a dead end, he took no further interest.

Stalemate. Lysenko had been banned, and the strange chapter seemed closed. Yet now, in an unlikely plot twist, Rodchenkov and Lysenko were standing before Vitaly. And Rodchenkov was talking about Lysenko competing in Beijing? Vitaly thought someone in a high place must be on Lysenko's side.

Coach Beloborodov had in fact raised the stakes. The International Association of Athletics Federations (IAAF), he claimed, would show clemency to his throwers if it was proven that they had indeed been duped by the former national coach. They might also cut their sentence to just one year if the women co-operated with the investigation. That is, if they named names. And with only a one-year ban in place they could go to Beijing.

'It's necessary to impose stricter sanctions on the former head coach [Kulichenko],' Beloborodov had elaborated. 'Certainly we're not ready, speaking in general terms, to sell out all of Russia. But concerning our concrete matter, we are ready to divulge all information, to describe everything that we know ... If they lay down their hands and won't fight for us, we will have to act further. We'll begin to ruin Kulichenko's system, which continues to function. To whom it concerns, they will understand what I'm talking about. We have a chance with the IAAF, and I'm certain it must be taken.'

Selling out Russia! Unfortunate accidents sometimes befell people who spoke this way. Beloborodov was either very confident or dangerously naive.

In these early days, people at Rusada would certainly have thought of Vitaly as naive, with all his talk of fighting doping. What they didn't understand was that Vitaly was also on first-name terms with pragmatism. He needed this job.

'Can you hurry, please?' Rodchenkov pressed him now. 'I need this sample.'

'Again, Dr Rodchenkov, she is a female and I am male. How am I supposed to do this?'

'She will just bring the sample to you. Fill out the doping control forms, seal the sample and give it all to me.'

His voice had a serrated edge that Vitaly found persuasive.

In the end Vitaly loitered outside the lavatory door until Lysenko emerged bearing her beaker of what seemed crystal-clear urine. He bagged and tagged the sample, brought it to Rodchenkov and knew that now he could no longer call himself pure. He went home and waited. For days and for weeks he worried. This would unravel and the sword would fall on him, just as it had on Kulichenko.

He told the entire story to Director Sinev, who said, 'Vitaly, relax.'

Chapter 3

Mid-August 2009, offices of Rusada
Another conversation between Vitaly and Director Sinev

'Director Sinev?'

'Vitaly. Come in. Come in. You look worried as usual, my friend.'

'No, not really. I just need to ask you something.'

'That's what I'm here for, I think!'

'Well, I know that you have holiday plans for the beginning of September.'

'Yes, yes. Time off for you from driving me around! I get a holiday and you get a little holiday too.'

'I was wondering if I could have some time off at that time too.'

'Well, it is sudden but it shouldn't be a problem. Leave it with me. Are you going anywhere special?'

'Remember that girl I told you about last week that I had a date with? She has competitions in Sochi at the beginning of September. Regional competitions, and then the next week they will stay by the beach and relax. It's the end of their season. Anyway, I would like to go with her. It is agreed between us.'

'Well okay, Vitaly, but I will say it again: be careful. You can't hurry love.'

~

Sometimes true love runs like a white-water ride.

The second date was much like the first. Yuliya was coming through Moscow to catch an onward flight, so Vitaly suggested they see each other. This time she defrosted a little more, but if you were a global-warming denier you would say, 'Look, no significant thaw.' She was scheduled to pass through Moscow on her way back, too and Vitaly, pushing hard, pressed his apartment key on her, gave her his address and urged her to stay at his place on her way home. She didn't demur.

A couple of days later she duly arrived, and so began their third date. She updated him on the process of getting to run for the police. Russia had changed but in its soul it was still the same. Tricky.

After clearing a medical examination, she would be registered for employment by the police. The venue and medical staff for the examination had to be approved by *militsiya*, as the police were then known. But two snags had cropped up: the doctors had decided that Yuliya was underweight, and the police required an X-ray of Yuliya's chest and lungs. This latter evidence had to be provided and paid for by Yuliya herself. Vitaly couldn't see where the difficulty lay. Yuliya certainly had a chest and lungs, so why didn't she just get an X-ray?

'Idiot. It's not so simple. I had tuberculosis.'

'When was this?'

'When I was still a student back in Kursk. I was in hospital for three months.'

He audited the available data on this woman. Dope cheat. Family trouble. Tuberculosis. An ailment of the poor.

'Would they be able to tell you've had tuberculosis?'

'Yes.'

'I see. So, what did you do?'

He was helplessly drawn towards her – her strength and her vulnerability, the darkness of her past against the promise of her future. There was something about her that he could feel but not define. Every word and gesture pulled him in.

'I needed somebody else's lungs.'

'A transplant?'

'No. Idiot.'

A few days after the first examination, she returned to the police doctor. She had forced the biggest meal of her life into her body. She had weights concealed on every part of her person. Desperate measures but they bought her a pass. Without comment the doctor ticked the box. Then, as cool as you like, she handed over an X-ray of two impeccable lungs. The label on the envelope said 'Yuliya Rusanova'. The doctor took the X-rays, held them up and nodded. Yes, all good.

The lungs belonged to her younger sister, Angelina, whom they called Gelia. She'd gone to the radiology department at Kursk hospital to present herself and her lungs for X-ray and had simply said, 'I'm Yuliya Rusanova and I have an appointment.' Russian bureaucracy was like a mountain range: some tunnelled through it inch by inch, but generally it was easier to just swerve around it.

Yuliya told Vitaly these things and he realised that she came from a different world with bigger troubles and harsher rules than he'd ever known.

She had been small as a kid. Life was poor·and tough in Kursk, but she ran fast. And speed was something she could make a career from. They noticed her and they told her that potential was just potential. In time they would sit her down and give her the talk. The rules. The facts of life. You want to get out of this dump of a city? You want to go to international competitions? You want to have an apartment and a car? You want to win things? Yes? Wise up, then. She absorbed their information and she took the decision on her own. She knew it was wrong. She also knew it was necessary.

'Is it fair or sporting or idealistic?' Vitaly would ask about the decision to dope.

'No,' she said. 'Is anything?'

He wanted to know where her cynicism came from. And so began a long conversation with just the two of them speaking softly about hard things.

Kursk. He knew nothing about the place apart from its inconvenient distance from Moscow. The biggest tank battle in history was fought in Kursk in 1943. The tanks they had built in Vitaly's home town, Chelyabinsk, had been blown apart in Kursk. A German general had written to Hitler.

'Do you think anyone even knows where Kursk is?'

Good question.

At the best of times there was little for a kid to do in Kursk, and the best of times had already passed by the time Yuliya hit her teens. After school she and Katia would clean the apartment, await the arrival of their mum and then brace themselves for whatever mood Igor would bring home. Igor drank in the parks or on the street. Usually he came home angry. He expressed frustration through his fists. Lyubov was the primary target but, as Yuliya, Katia and Gelia grew, Igor blamed them too. They would run to shield their mother. He would get a few oaths and punches in before they backed down. Yuliya thought he hated them all, that he hated their loyalty to each other, their closeness. And her dad knew that they hated him. Especially Yuliya.

∼

For years Yuliya's escape was to Tutova, the village where she had lived as a child with her maternal grandparents. The love they swaddled her in, the swing Grandpa Mikhail had built just for her, the ritual of picking strawberries or mushrooms with Grandma Nadia. Everything about Tutova was better that Kursk.

After her family's time in the nature reserve came to an end, Yuliya was farmed out to one set of grandparents, Katia to the other. Yuliya stayed at Tutova until she was seven. Happy times. There were animals and even a few pets. Cows, horses, pigs, chickens. Tutova was a hamlet, maybe twenty houses, each subsisting on its own plot of land as Tutova families had always done. In the summer Yuliya gathered strawberries. There was sunshine and she had red juice on her lips. In autumn they went to the forest to pick mushrooms. Grandma marinated the mushrooms in vinegar and sealed them in jars to be stored for the winter.

How her parents actually came to loan out their children is another story. Lyubov and Igor had three daughters, which for Igor constituted one disappointment after another. Three girls when he yearned for a son. Three mouths were too many. After the nature reserve, Igor and Lyubov went to work in a rubber factory. The money was a little better but not enough. Never enough. So they kept little Gelia and loaned out the older two.

In the city Igor worked hard and drank hard, but when the family went to the country he found happiness in the soil. He grew vegetables and on summer evenings and holidays Igor, Lyubov and their daughters came together and worked a little strip of Russia they could call their own. They grew potatoes, carrots, cabbage. Anything they could. What they didn't eat they sold at the farmers' market. The money bought clothes for Katia, which would be passed down, frayed and familiar, to Yuliya. When Yuliya outgrew the clothes, Gelia was ready to grow into them.

Nothing in the city gave Igor the same pride as the land offered him. The girls too preferred the countryside, even if they weren't as devoted to the vegetable plot as their dad.

Working the vegetable garden didn't compare with being coddled by Grandpa Mikhail, who would dance comically for Yuliya when she was bored or cranky. She was his favourite. Years later she would look back on those times as golden.

Igor kept beehives too and the process of extracting honey from patient labour absorbed him. His face filled with pride and wonder as he held up a jar of honey from his own hives. In the daytime in the city he was another drone in a rubber factory. In Tutova, though, he supervised the production of thousands of busy workers. In those moments he wasn't the bitter soak that they came to dread.

Now, when Yuliya wants to think of the best times with her dad, she remembers the honey and what it meant to him.

~

The earlier conversation about other relationships? Yuliya needed to revisit that. For clarity. She should have mentioned, she said now, that she was 'kind of in a relationship' with her coach.

'Kind of in a relationship?'

'Yeah. Kind of crazy. He has a family. He has a daughter. He has grandchildren even.'

'Really? Are you making fun of me?'

She wasn't. Her coach had promised he would leave them all and that they would get married. For a time she believed him. She understood now though that the lie was his way of hand-cuffing her to him. She knew that marriage was never going to happen. He would never leave his wife.

'And?'

'Nothing. It's just a lie he's been telling. That's all.'

Vitaly was astonished by how quickly he found himself to be in love. This girl. He had never met anybody so fractured yet so tough and strong. Her indifference intrigued him.

28

She laid everything out so bluntly. Take it or leave it. Mostly he took it.

Suppose she met somebody, he thought, *and, without her realising it, this somebody was 'the one'?* Suppose she could wake up some day with the sun coming through a high window and just lie there, feeling warm and safe and happy. She would look across at the man sleeping beside her and know that he had always loved her. She'd smile at how he had persisted, undeterred by her toughness or her suspicion. She would be happy in a way she never thought possible.

Or suppose she just doesn't give a shit. Suppose she sees you as an amusement, a convenience store on the highway between Kursk and wherever. Suppose she talks about you to her coach, her lover, when she goes home to Kursk: This doping control guy, he gives me lifts and buys me food and lets me stay with him and I don't even have to pretend to him about anything.

This was their third date. She was in his Moscow apartment, fascinating him and tormenting him. There was something he needed to ask before he could let things go any further.

Chapter 4

A time pre-Rusada

When Vitaly had arrived in Moscow three years previously, he stayed briefly with Faya, a sister of his maternal grandmother. Faya lived with her son Igor in an apartment to the north of the city. In her mid- to late seventies, Faya was the woman for whom the word 'babushka' was invented. Igor was clinging to the hopeful side of fifty. Then cupid blindsided Igor. Suddenly, in the autumn of his unremarkable years, he was in love. In the little Moscow apartment, Vitaly was now in the way.

Vitaly understood. He moved out. He paid his rent by holding down a series of jobs until his luck changed. Which it eventually did.

Vitaly met Olga. An apartment that Vitaly's parents owned in Moscow was suddenly vacated by the tenants. Vitaly courted the girl and claimed the living space. It was an upturn but he still needed to upgrade his job if Olga was to be kept in the style that she felt to be her entitlement.

He had been a volunteer worker at the EuroLeague Final Four basketball games in May 2005. He hadn't been in Moscow for long and it was glamorous. CSKA, the big dogs of Russian hoops, had lost the semi-final to the Basques of Tau Cerámica. Vitaly viewed the weekend as an opportunity to let CSKA personnel know that he was available for hire. CSKA had two attractions: wages and Sergey Kushchenko.

Kushchenko was a genius. He had founded the Ural Great basketball club with his friend Andrey Vatutin. In 2001 and 2002 Ural Great had won the league, breaking the monopoly enjoyed by CSKA. The hicks from the sticks had surpassed the great club of the Russian Army.

This was the new Russia. Things had changed. You didn't always have to make your enemies vanish. Now you could buy them. Kushchenko and Vatutin were lured to Moscow and asked to make CSKA great again. A few years later bailiffs were in the Molot Sports Hall in Perm, sifting the wreckage of Ural Great's financial collapse. Kushchenko gave lectures on the Sports Management course that Vitaly was taking. Occasionally Vitaly would corner the great man and earnestly thrust his CV into his hands. You never knew. A year after the 2005 Final Four tournament was over, CSKA called.

Vitaly's monthly income more than doubled, to $1,000 a month. He liked the work and the people. He translated contracts, cleared paperwork, made himself useful. Best of all, he became part of the famous pick-up matches that Kushchenko and his circle played twice a week. Vitaly slotted in as a dogged defence man amid the showboating, slam-dunking executives. A steal here, a block there, the odd rebound and a talent for starting attacks from deep in the court were good enough to get Vitaly promoted from the opposition to a spot on Kushchenko's side. Then one evening, with a game going to the wire, Vitaly made a steal, burst out of a pivot and, on the bounce, let the ball hop just out of bounds. He stopped and tossed the ball to an opponent.

'Out of bounds,' he said with a shake of his head, making the call on himself. Nobody else had noticed. Kushchenko issued a cold glance as he passed.

'You're not a team player, Vitaly.'

Then there was the blog. In Soviet times information was drip-fed to the proletariat via *Pravda*, the Communist Party newspaper, and *Izvestia*, the state newspaper. *Pravda* translated into English as 'The Truth'. *Izvestia* was 'The News'. People said that there was no truth in the news and no news in the truth. Long before Donald Trump, Russians were aware of fake news. Russia's new, post-Soviet media found it difficult to shake off old habits. Objective voices were hard to find and often seemed to have a short career expectancy or, in a few cases, a short life expectancy.

Vitaly was analytical by nature. He liked to dismantle a subject and then put it back together again, having examined every facet. Like many young people in the new Russia, he blogged. He wrote mainly about sport and avoided politics but there were times when those worlds intersected. For example, when Vladimir Putin announced in 2007 that he would not be running for a third consecutive term as president as it would have been unconstitutional, the only people who didn't smell a rat were those who'd lost their sense of smell.

Putin would create the illusion of a contest for the presidency he was vacating. Just like in a real democracy. The public would appear to elect a placeholder – Dmitry Medvedev or Sergei Ivanov – and Putin would become prime minister. Four years later Putin would be free to become president again. The placeholder president was going to be one of the good old boys from Putin's St Petersburg past. Medvedev ultimately got Putin's nod, but for a while Ivanov's more conservative background had made him look like a better bet.

Vitaly blogged about the implications of Ivanov – a keen backer of CSKA and a constant presence at basketball games – becoming president of Russia. Some time later Vitaly's mentor, Kushchenko, moved higher up the CSKA ladder. His direct replacement was his old Ural Great partner, Andrey Vatutin, who had actually given Vitaly his chance with CSKA. Now he summoned Vitaly to his office.

'A CSKA staff member should not mention anything to do with this organisation in a personal blog,' Vatutin said. And now he regretted that there was no longer a job for Vitaly.

'Noted. Maybe you could give me another chance,' Vitaly said.

Vatutin paused then said, 'No.'

A while later, on New Year's Eve, Vitaly picked up a freesheet in a grocery store. He scanned the work ads.

'Degree necessary.' No.

'Experience necessary.' No.

'Candidate should be prepared to . . .' No.

'Applicants should have . . .' No.

'Staff wanted for new doping control agency.' Go back. What was that last one?

He posted a CV the next day. Things moved fast. A call. An interview. The state was creating a Russian anti-doping agency in accordance with the WADA code. Young people were needed who wanted to work in this kind of organisation.

They had found one such person. He began working at Rusada on 1 February 2008.

Chapter 5

Sometimes when she was still young and they were back in Kursk, Yuliya would ask her father why he lived as he did. She remembered his honey bees and his high hopes. Now he had his alcohol and nothing else.

'Why do you live like this, Papa?'

'Live like this? Me? Well, your mother is not easy. She raises a stink every day. You know what I mean by raise a stink? I work hard all day and then your mother is another day's work.'

Yuliya had hoped for more. She said nothing.

In the first few years of the new Russia, if your boat had been lifted on the tide you were given the chance to forget. You forgot the old Russia with its damp grey queues. You forgot those black jokes.

'What is 200 feet long and eats vegetables?'

'A queue for meat in Leningrad.'

'Knock-knock.'

'Who's there?'

'Your neighbour from downstairs. Get out, get out quick. The whole building is on fire.'

'Thank God. We thought it was the police.'

The Rusanovs couldn't forget. When Russia opened the sluices to Western money, barely a dribble reached Kursk. Men still drank cheap liquor in streets and parks. People fought and people killed each other. The police never came for fighting. For a murder sometimes they showed up. Moscow with its oligarchs, swish foreigners and coffee franchises was another country.

The Rusanovs lived in the cheapest part of a cheap city. Kursk's history was about endurance. Endurance was affordable but, like the cheap alcohol, it rotted you from the inside. Lyubov and Igor endured together. They worked in the same factory, making car tyres in bad light. The smell of rubber clung to them and they came to hate the factory, just as they grew to hate each other. As Igor saw it, 'Why do you live like this?' was a dumb question for Yuliya to ask him. The question was *how*? 'How do you live like this, Papa?' He didn't know the answer to that.

Grandpa Mikhail had retired from his life as a small farmer but he kept pigs to be killed and occasionally a calf nursed from birth would be brought to town for somebody else to buy and to slaughter. The proceeds went into Lyubov's purse, Grandpa's way of helping his daughter and his grandchildren. Yuliya never mourned those skinny, docile cows. Their slaughter brought money. When a cow had been traded Yuliya would ask her mother if she might buy her some clothes.

'I have no money,' Lyubov would say. Nothing more, but Yuliya knew she was lying.

Eventually Yuliya figured it out. Lyubov kept it all under the bed, accumulating slowly. The more the pile of money grew, the more Yuliya resented her mother. Why save for a rainy day when you are already drowning?

Her father, meanwhile, grew more problematic. After work he would meet with friends. They bought alcohol in stores and sat in the park and drank. A confederacy of sour drunks. Sometimes they drank vodka. More often they drank samogon, the cheap moonshine that was the drink of choice for the poor. Samogon was made by your friends or friends of your friends.

It was dirt cheap and it made you mad. In some places it outsold vodka by five to one despite being the bottled version of Russian roulette. Anything from dimedrol to methanol might be added for effect. You never knew what you were drinking, just that you were getting drunk. Igor liked samogon.

Yuliya's earliest memory of her dad's drinking was from a night in the little fourth-floor apartment in Kursk. She was almost asleep. Her mother had been home from work for a few hours. Igor arrived home from the park. He was noisy and it was already late. She knew by the sounds he made that he was drunk but she closed her eyes and tried to sleep. They were fighting, though. She could hear all the shouting and then her mother crying and then an ambulance came. Yuliya was eight years old and crying and standing in pyjamas. Igor had taken a heavy box and hit her mother in the head with it.

For as long as Yuliya could remember, Uncle Anatoly never spoke to his sister Lyubov. That was a fact of life and there were bigger things for an eight-year-old girl to worry about. Now she recalled her mother telling her that her father had once come home from the factory drunk as usual. His mood was unusually foul and when he set about attacking Lyubov, Grandma Nadia had tried to protect her daughter. Igor had pushed her violently and Nadia had fallen hard onto an old bicycle that leaned against a wall. A pedal or a handlebar – nobody was ever too sure which – punched hard into her side. The hospital said that the damage was to her liver, and X-rays showed an ominously large and dark spot on the organ. Some months later Nadia died from liver failure. She was in her mid-fifties. Cancer of the liver was the official cause of death, but Uncle Anatoly had always believed that Igor had killed his mother.

From that night when the ambulance had come, Yuliya knew no peace. The curtain came down on her childhood. Her father drank more and he drank worse. If Lyubov wasn't there when he came home, he picked on his daughters. If Lyubov was there, the little girls ran to protect her and absorbed the brunt of his anger.

'My sisters and I, every time we tried to save our mum,' Yuliya says to Vitaly, holding on to the part she can bear to remember.

Not that she wasn't scared of her dad. When he came for her it was like war. She grew used to it and if anything she grew more defiant, but long after he was gone the bad dreams lingered. The end, when it arrived, didn't come in their apartment in Kursk but in the little village where she had enjoyed her happiest times.

Yuliya told Vitaly things that, to her, were run-of-the-mill stuff, scenes of everyday life in her corner of Kursk. No drama, no casting herself as victim, no plea for sympathy. This is how it was, and it wasn't all bad.

When she was seventeen, she'd discovered running and begun training in athletics. Nothing very serious but she discovered after a stretch of training that she was improving, that she could run faster. She liked that. It encouraged her to believe that a life beyond Kursk was possible. She wanted to run like a professional. Professional athletes made money and didn't live in Kursk. She didn't know where precisely they lived – Moscow probably – but she decided to train every day regardless. By now she had accepted that her father would never again be that happy man with his jar full of honey. When marinating in samogon, his seed turned bad.

In the lengthening days of spring and the long days of summer, her father would order her to the village to work in the fields. She said that she couldn't and she wouldn't because she had to train. His hatred for her grew every time she defied him. She gave the hatred right back to him. Toe to toe, eye to eye. From defiance she drew strength, and the stronger she grew the better she ran. *Keep it coming*, she thought, *keep it coming*.

She was in training camp when it happened.

Igor went to the village alone and fell into drinking with Grandpa Mikhail. Both men were alcoholics but Grandpa Mikhail was an easy and lovable drunk. Nobody ever knew the details of what exactly occurred but in the morning Lyubov phoned Yuliya at training camp and told her that she needed to come home. Grandpa Mikhail was dead. Igor had beaten Grandpa to death with the stout stick that the old man used for mashing pig feed.

Yuliya was happy when her father went to prison. He would never come home to them again. There would be no more wars. He sat in prison for seven years and they had a rest from him. Lyubov divorced him without any trouble. Her sisters visited their father in prison from time to time but Yuliya never went. She never wrote and she never asked about him. Maybe it was different for Katia and Gelia. She didn't spend much time wondering about why they went to see him. At night she still had the nightmares about him. So did Lyubov. That was their inheritance.

She kept running obsessively.

Vitaly was excited to see that she loved to run. He smiled to himself and allowed a playful thought to linger: Mr and Mrs Forrest Gump! But he knew that she saw things not quite as he did.

Some people, seldom Russians, spoke mystically about the sensation of running, the endorphins, the clear-headedness, the energy, the feathery lightness, the chi of it. For Yuliya it was simpler: running was a ticket to a better life. She understood clearly that she could make money on a track. Her family never had money and knew nobody who could get her onto the ladder that would lead to a good job. Yuliya would have to make her own way. If the speed at which she ran could help to pay for better things then she would do whatever it took to get faster.

The 800 metres was a race of maximum pain. Two laps, flat

out. When the body wept with pain there was still 250 metres left to run. It wasn't a case of who could inflict the most pain but who could endure the most. She was good with that deal. Your legs hurt? Your chest hurts? That's not real pain. She had Kursk in her being. She could endure more than most.

When Igor died she surprised herself. For a while, she wept every day. She would remember her dad in the fields. And she would recall the two occasions that she went to meet him after he got out of prison. Once, they had sat across a table from each other, talking awkwardly as they ate. She hadn't been sure who this person was or if she had anything left to offer to him. He had been pale and a little fatter than she remembered him but better in himself than before. Calmer. Drinking just a little, he had said. She'd told him that if he started drinking again she would not have a father. Never. And if he started a new life and tried to be a good man she might have a father and she would talk to him. He had been quiet. He'd had nothing to say. No promises to make. That was all.

When he was in prison Igor had stopped smoking because blood came up when he coughed and he was afraid of dying in prison. Free again, he had gone back to tobacco. He died from lung cancer at fifty-two. As much as her life would change, Yuliya's memories stayed with her. Grandpa Mikhail waiting for her, being happy to see her. The good times before it all went wrong.

Vitaly listened to her story, soaking it up. This small, beautiful woman and her fucked-up, broken life. She was more moonlight than sunlight.

And she doped.

And there was still a question he needed to ask.

Chapter 6

After a slow beginning, new recruits arrived at Rusada and were assigned to desks, and suddenly there were enough people to justify meetings being held. The office on Kazakova Street became a hive. Everybody worked in a second-floor room designed for half as many people. To make things worse, the newly appointed doping control officers used the place between missions, collecting kits and documentation, spreading the pollen of gossip as they came and went.

Director Sinev managed it all from a room down on the first floor. He worked alongside Aleksandr Derevoedov, the head of the medical department. Derevoedov was in the process of bedding into the new organisation. He had helped set up Rusada but he still drew his wage from Rossport, the Federal Agency for Physical Education and Sports. It was Derevoedov who had recruited Sinev and who had rubber-stamped Vitaly's employment. He mattered.

In March a guy called Igor Zagorskiy joined. His was a grandiose title, Head of International Communications. Zagorskiy was the same age as Vitaly, young with a lank mullet of dark hair. Despite the title, his job was mostly translation work. If Sinev or Derevoedov went to an anti-doping conference Zagorskiy tagged along and did the translating. Rusada's engagement with other countries and other national anti-doping organisations pleased Vitaly. He too could translate, but it was thick documents and dry protocols that filled his days.

In the spring some people from WADA arrived, descending like a small flock of high-flying diplomats. They had good suits, white teeth and they were earnest and encouraging. They shook hands firmly and spoke of upcoming conferences. Rob Koehler, head of the education department, was there, as was the agency's European director, Jean-Pierre Moser, and people from Finnish Anti-Doping who would provide doping control officer training for Rusada's young staff, including Vitaly. The visitors wanted to see that everything was good. And what wasn't to admire about Russia setting up its own anti-doping agency?

By the summer of 2008 the new agency was gaining traction. The office hummed as the first sample collection operations loomed. It felt like mission control for a space launch.

Vitaly was by now providing doping control training for eight raw Rusada recruits who had arrived with no experience. The other eight doping control officers had been transferred from Rossport and were set in their ways. The eight whom Vitaly trained were as eager as the other eight were cynical. The future of Rusada seemed to hinge on which group would have the most influence. Those who'd come from the Federal Agency seemed to know more and care less, enduring the presence of the new recruits but not thinking much of Vitaly's hard-to-fathom idealism.

There was one former doping control officer from the Federal Agency who'd lost his job and felt more than a little put out. In the field of anti-doping he was a minor celebrity as he communicated openly with the federations in advance of his doping control missions. He liked to be open with them and his transparency stretched to informing all interested parties about who he hoped to take samples from and what exactly those samples might be tested for. He would ask warmly where everybody was going to socialise with him later on. He had taken the changes badly. He had heard about Vitaly, and called him on the phone, drunk and bitter.

'You are young, and you don't understand anything. You are not doing things the right way. This is Russia and this is not the way it works in Russia. You just don't understand. It will come against you.'

Vitaly listened as his failings were enumerated. He was naive. He was wrong-headed. He was going to spoil things for everybody. Who did he think he was, messing with people's livelihoods? Would he be thanked? No, he would not. He should watch out.

'Thank you for all that,' said Vitaly. 'Goodbye.'

Vitaly went to find Sinev and Derevoedov and told them of the phone call. He was met with smiles all round. The usual gentle rebuff.

'Don't worry, Vitaly. You're such a worrier!'

More calls came. Vitaly listened and did what he had been told. He didn't worry.

Mostly the work was dispiriting. Anti-doping codes and protocols that needed to be translated from English into Russian, though he seemed to do more editing than translating. The English-language codes shrunk in translation. WADA's book of doping control protocols lost key parts. The manual for DCOs went from being an eighty-page document in English to being a slender ten-page pamphlet in Russian. Derevoedov's inspections inevitably led to more watering-down of the rules.

'Ah Vitaly, look at this . . . sometimes this is not possible to do in Russia.' He'd run his finger over a large tract of WADA text. 'So we can take all this stuff out. It's not for us.'

Another day: 'Vitaly, I think the Russian doping control officer can be more flexible than his international counterpart, no? So let's take this out and take this out and change this part.'

Brevity. Flexibility. The acceptance that all things are not possible in Russia.

For Vitaly, the launch of Rusada's testing missions couldn't come quickly enough. In the meantime, there was the excitement of another visit from some important people from WADA in May. Stuart Kemp, operations manager, flew in behind the main posse, and Rusada sent Vitaly to collect him at the airport. They say that a drive in Moscow is like a Communist Party speech: it seldom takes less than three hours and doesn't get you very far. The journey gave Vitaly and Stuart time to get to know each other.

The young driver had a useful personality quirk: he actually enjoyed the traffic. He drove a Toyota Caldina, a Japanese car with the steering wheel on the right side – a detail that appeared to have escaped Vitaly's notice as he pulled confidently into the oncoming traffic, staring down approaching drivers. In the passenger seat Kemp felt as if he'd put his life in the hands of a Russian who didn't much value it. He was wrong, though. Vitaly enjoyed the presence of the WADA people. He hoped that they would convert his Russian colleagues to the cause of anti-doping.

Kemp asked questions. Vitaly's answers were honest and unusually heartfelt. Beneath the Russian eccentricities, Kemp could see a young man who cared about anti-doping. If this was the calibre of employee at Rusada, Russia wasn't in a bad place. By the time they arrived at Rusada's office, a bond had developed.

Not long after the WADA visit, Director Sinev and Vitaly sat opposite each other at Sinev's desk.

'Beijing,' said Sinev, not making it clear whether it was a statement or a question.

'What about it?' asked Vitaly.

Stuart Kemp had, apparently, returned to WADA, where he had fallen into a conversation with one Stacy Spletzer. Neither Vitaly or Director Sinev had ever heard of this Stacy Spletzer but hers was a name spangled with North American promise. Spletzer was setting up WADA Outreach teams for the Beijing

Games. She felt it would be a good move to have a Russian presence on Outreach. Somebody young and enthusiastic who spoke English fluently and who could talk about the educational part of anti-doping. She'd asked if Kemp had come across anybody.

'Would he have to drive people anywhere?' Kemp had asked. 'No? Then I think I may have just the person.'

Sinev beamed paternally as he bestowed the gift of Beijing on his protégé.

'Beijing, then?'

'Beijing!' said Vitaly.

The first thought racing into his head was: *Call home. Tell your parents their son not only has a job but he's off to the Olympics. He's living his dream.* The second thought was that dreams should be tested for snags before their owner signs off on them.

Vitaly's foreign passport had expired in 2005. Getting a new passport was more complicated than photo booths, forms and queues. More complicated than just dropping roubles into the right policeman's mitt. In October 1967, when Russia was a different country, the Duma had decreed that any male citizen could be drafted into the army once he had reached the age of eighteen. Russian males turning seventeen found their names registered in the military directory or *voinskii uchet*. They were eligible to be drafted until the age of twenty-seven.

Vitaly had just turned twenty-six. When he applied for a passport his name would pop up on the *voinskii uchet*. Mother Russia would demand twelve months of his time. And that would be the end of Beijing.

Chapter 7

In late June 2008 Vitaly went on a testing mission with Irina Verbitskaya, another doping control officer. Rusada booked them flights to Vitaly's home town of Chelyabinsk. The National Junior Athletic Championships would be a three-day assignment.

Vitaly told Irina a story from earlier in June when he'd been working at the national freestyle wrestling championships in St Petersburg. The contact for doping control in the wrestling federation had arrived in a Porsche Cayenne. Mr Porsche approached Vitaly and the accompanying DCO, offering them about $50 worth of cash each.

'Guys. Here's cash to go out in the evenings. Make sure you have money for drinks and a good time.'

Irina, the other DCO, a woman who'd come from the Federal Agency, looked mournfully at Mr Porsche.

'We can't do that any more,' she said.

'Whatever,' said Mr Porsche and he took his money and left.

Vitaly shook his head solemnly. Irina's hopes of a good night out in Chelyabinsk had just died. As Vitaly had intended them to.

On the second day in Chelyabinsk the women's 400 metres final took place. A coach hurried to the doping control area immediately after the race and spoke to Irina.

'Look, we should do this in the way we used to do it. My girl just won. It's better if you don't take the sample. Can you take somebody else's? Like the old days?'

'Speak to Vitaly,' said Irina.

Vitaly heard out the request. 'No,' he said.

The coach asked again, more insistently.

'There is nothing to discuss,' said Vitaly. 'She won. Now we must test her.'

Now the vice president of the Russian Athletics Federation joined the conversation to add the weight of his office.

'Come,' he said to Vitaly, 'let's go to VIP room.' The vice president seemed quite drunk. 'Look, we cannot test this athlete. Okay? How much money do you want?'

The vice president waved his wallet.

'I don't need money,' Vitaly replied.

This news was taken calmly.

'If there is not enough in my wallet I can give you more. Just tell me how much.'

'Really, there is nothing to talk about.'

Vitaly left. From the doping control area he called Director Sinev in Moscow.

'Okay, Vitaly,' Sinev reflected. 'Thank you for telling me.'

The athlete arrived in doping control and sat there, rehydrating herself until she could provide a sample. The atmosphere was strained. The phone rang. It was Sinev.

'Don't test her.'

'What?'

'Don't test her, but make sure you tell them this is the last time.'

'Really?'

'Yes.'

Vitaly climbed down.

The next day was the 4 × 400 metres relay. A random selection saw the same girl get picked.

'Shit,' said Vitaly.

She turned up at doping control, though. Alone. No complaints. Everything normal. *Well*, thought Vitaly, *I may have made my point.*

Back in Moscow he spoke to Director Sinev, who was as affable and evasive as always.

'Just don't worry so much, Vitaly.'

Later he learned the truth. New procedures had been put in place for that Sunday. If the 400 metres athlete needed to give another sample, the instruction was to just do it and send the code number to the laboratory. It would be taken care of. No need to involve the pesky middleman from Rusada. If you thought about it, this was progress for the coach and his athlete. A new, streamlined protocol.

Vitaly was compiling his own personal anthology of in-the-field stories. Evidence, you could say. He didn't know who he would ever show these exhibits to but he gathered them in hope. Other testers were happy to just hit the numbers. If the samples never got checked or the rules weren't followed, why worry? Tests were being done. Money was coming in. Rusada was doing its job. There were graphs and tables and stats to prove it.

Vitaly always returned to Moscow full of woe and offering Director Sinev his latest weary tale. It didn't matter how much hostility he encountered in the field, he kept on. The next mission, the next tests. The equipment he carried felt heavier with each outing.

You prepare for a mission. First rule: always bring enough equipment. Kits, kits, kits. Each Bereg-Kit was packed in a cardboard box sealed in printed shrink-wrap. Each kit was uniquely numbered on all the components: cardboard box, bottles and security caps.

You will have: *Clean, sealed urine collection vessels. Partial sample kits. Equipment for measuring specific gravity. Sealed, tamper-proof bottles/containers for A and B samples. Each Bereg-Kit contains two glass bottles, one A-bottle (orange), one B-bottle (blue), both with a security cap and sealed with a shrink-sleeve wrap. Secure courier transport bags/containers. Disposable gloves providing barrier protection. Soap, handwash or anti-bacterial gel/liquid. Paper towels or other absorbent material. Garbage bin/bags. Individually sealed non-alcoholic beverages. Scissors, pens and other applicable stationery. All Doping Control documentation including Doping Control forms, athlete notification forms (if not part of the Doping Control form), supplementary report forms, Chain of Custody forms, DCO report forms, etc. Any other equipment specified by the relevant laboratory.*

It was a lot of trouble for so little respect.

Exhibit B

The track cycling championships were held at the Sports Center of Trade Unions in Krylatskoye, a district of Moscow. Vitaly was head DCO. Months ago he had written to every national federation. 'Hello. We are Rusada. We are the good guys. Trust us. Please let us know the person responsible for anti-doping in your federation. Yours in sport, Thank you.' Some federations never replied, but Vitaly persisted and his contacts list had grown.

The contacts were expected to help with the recruitment of chaperones and to facilitate the testing. Cycling's anti-doping officer was ready to make things very straightforward. He handed a list of names to Vitaly.

'All these competitors are clean.'

'Okay, but we still do random selection.'

'No. No need. They are clean, for sure.'

'Clean for sure? Good! If they are selected, they'll have no worries.'

This didn't go down well. Silence, tinged with surliness, followed. Vitaly was about to move on to the question of chaperones but before he could—

'If that is how you want it,' interrupted the cycling officer, 'I won't help you at all at championships. You do it yourself.'

'If you don't want to help, that is fine.'

It wasn't fine. Anything but. Track cycling is like party games for very fit people on very expensive bikes. Each event seemed more confusing than the one before. Vitaly watched a match sprint. It should be straightforward, one-on-one, the winner is whoever is first over the line, so surely he goes through? Not so. And this was the most straightforward event he saw.

Three-man time trials were held over three laps with teams starting on opposite sides of the track. After the end of each lap, the leading rider pulled off completely. Where the hell did he go? Pursuits were worse. Two four-man teams started on opposite sides of the track. Something called the keirin was paced by a motorbike leading out a field of eight riders. And the madison. What the . . . ? A mass start of two-man teams but after a while only one rider from each team could be on the track at any time. The changeovers were hair-raising. Then the omnium. More craziness.

Vitaly would have needed a platoon of former KGB goons just to track down the people he wanted to test. When a race finished, nobody knew for some time who the winner was. Mostly they milled about on the track but some cycled off for warm-downs and others disappeared into the ant colony on the infield. And everybody wore helmets. Vitaly had no chaperones. But this was the game. If you want to do your tests, you do them our way.

~

The army gathered up its draftees twice a year, in spring and autumn. Few young Russians went willingly. In the wind-whipped hells to which young men were dispatched, the oldest recruits, the *stariki*, ritually bullied the fresh kids. This was the old army tradition of *dedovshchina* or grandfathering. In 2006 there were 3,500 cases of *dedovshchina* recorded, but most cases were never reported. Extreme hazing. Beyond bullying. Malnutrition. Deprivation. Sexual abuse. Rape. Enslavement. Death. That was the deal with grandfathering.[1] It was often more frightening to be a Russian soldier in peacetime than in wartime.

There were many ways of avoiding the draft. If you officially received a notification, you were drafted. If you avoided receipt you would not be drafted. The simplest remedy? Hide. Otherwise fake an illness, maim yourself or forge some documents. If you could afford it, a prolonged college career was a popular option. Russia was dotted with private diploma mills where young men could study for PhDs until the threat of conscription went away on their twenty-seventh birthday. Whichever way you chose, you found the right person and bribed them. Doctors, college registrars, militia. Right up to the bribes of last resort: army men and draft board officials. Just about any idiot could avoid the draft. Unless the idiot needed to officially request a new passport.

Vitaly was cornered, screwed, *besperspektivnyak*.

In Russia, when you sit and assess the usefulness of everybody that you know and everybody that they know and then everybody that those people know, you no longer have friends and acquaintances, you have a network. That's called *blat*. Connections, pull, influence with a side order of nepotism. *Blat*.

Vitaly called Alexey, his friend from home. Bingo. Alexey's father knew the main military person in the district. Vitaly was told to go to him soon and give him a fat envelope. The correct papers with the correct stamp would materialise. Vitaly flew to Chelyabinsk at the first opportunity. Going to the District Army Office, he brought his dad along as wingman. There was only one guy on duty. The trick was to say nothing explicit. The army guy would know what was going down.

Or maybe not. As he spoke, Vitaly realised that the signals were all wrong. The *blat* wasn't working. This wasn't the man but he did direct the Stepanovs to the building next door where a sturdy woman was seated right at the entrance.

'Yes,' she said, 'and who are you?'

'Vitaly Stepanov.'

'Stepanov? Okay. Wait just a minute.'

Hallelujah. She knew the dance.

She wrote rapidly on a page on her desk and then handed the paper to Vitaly with a smile. *How perfectly choreographed our national corruption service is*, he thought.

'Thank you.'

'No, thank you,' she said, 'for your service.'

She had handed him a formal document of notification. Roughly it said, 'GO TO THE ARMY. Go directly to the Army. Do not pass Go. Do not collect Olympic accreditation. Do not go to Beijing.' If he signed the paper, he would be drafted. If he ran away, he would have committed a criminal offence.

'Dad,' he said, 'can I speak to you outside?'

Exhibit C

Vitaly went with a female colleague to test female weightlifters. Fish in a barrel for an anti-doping agency. Or so you would think. There was an old joke about the clean and jerk division: lots of jerks, very few cleans. Stretching back to Soviet days, there was a mighty culture of doped athletes who lifted heavy things or threw heavy things.

A national coach, Vladimir Ilyin, once pointed out that volunteers at doping control were often just that: volunteers. If they were offered some money they would do whatever they were asked. He added with a twinkle, 'I'm not talking about those who work in doping control in Russia or the former USSR. It's enough to offer them a nice meal.' He continued, 'In all the time I worked with the national team there was never an instance when I did not know the results of a test several days before they were on the desk of the head of the doping commission.'

They were incorrigible. Unremarkably, Russian weightlifters struggled at properly tested international competitions. Russia had one gold to show from the Sydney and Athens Games despite achieving fine results between Olympiads. So, carrying a list of athletes to be tested, Vitaly and his colleague drove to the training camp of the female weightlifters of Russia. Driving in was like a first glimpse of Jurassic Park. Small herds of bulked-up, power-loaded women roamed in their tracksuits. Any one of them capable of throwing Vitaly and perhaps his car back over the perimeter wall if they took against him.

He located the coach responsible for liaising with doping control. He seemed amused by Vitaly's presumption.

'You are here to test ten of our athletes?'

'That's right. Where should I set up?'

'Well, the first problem is that we only have four or five athletes here today.'

'That is a joke, right? I saw at least ten as I came up from the gate.'

'No, you didn't.'

'Yes, I did.'

'You do know that this is weightlifting?'

He explained it as if Vitaly was a child. Weightlifting. Most lifters are at a certain stage of their preparation and so they are not available for testing. They should be recorded as absent. Four or five lifters at a different stage of preparation would provide samples.

'Send me the four "who are here",' said Vitaly, 'and we'll go through the motions with them.'

Back in the office he told Sinev, Zagorskiy and Derevoedov. They thanked him for bringing this to their attention. They would be sure to write to the Federation.

Exhibit D

Vitaly was random-testing a baseball team, and half of that team was supposed to be present. Vitaly would appear and announce himself. Surprise! The players arrived late. After Vitaly had arrived. They looked like a baseball team from central casting. Chewing and spitting and joshing.

Vitaly and his sidekick said hello and began the process. Checking photos from the passports against the faces of the players. Hmm. None of the baseball players looked like the photographs in the passports they handed over. Not even close. It would be normal in one or two cases. Old pictures. Different hairstyles. Facial hair. A few bad snaps. But not a single face matched a photo. The supply of ringers wasn't even executed cleverly. Oh. They actually were all from central casting.

Vitaly was surprised that Russia even had baseball teams. Even more surprised that they went to the trouble of doping and sending ringers to tests. He called Sinev.

'What do we do?'

'Just leave.'

These matters were a numbers problem for Rusada, not an ethics problem. If an officer was dispatched to collect twelve samples but collected none then that created a deficit. The next mission would need to deliver extra samples and that's how Rusada muddled along, doing what it could to hit the numbers. That was the imperative. Bottom line. For every completed doping control form, Rusada collected 8,000 roubles. Targeting? Strategy? Testing for the right things at the right time? That was somebody else's worry.

The 'big misunderstanding' would take too much unraveling. Apologies flowed but really, what could be done? You went to the draft office with a bribe and you got drafted? Well . . .

The next morning Vitaly rose early and left the house without speaking to his parents. He took public transportation back to the District Army Office. Outside the army office there was a playground. Vitaly sat on a swing. He rocked slowly and watched the comings and goings. He sat for an hour, an hour and a half, and then rose and left. He had given fate its opening. Nobody from the army office had come to drag him to the barracks. He flew back to Moscow to wait for the ominous knock on his door.

And then later it hit him. *Blat.* Everybody you know. Everybody you ever knew. Of *course*. CSKA basketball club had cut him loose but he still had friends at CSKA, and CSKA was the traditional Red Army club. Of course.

He called a guy, a manager who liaised with the army people on behalf of the sports club. A schmoozer, a facilitator. He told the guy what he needed.

'No problem,' the guy said. 'One phone call and 10,000 roubles into a certain hand by tomorrow afternoon, Vitaly.'

'10,000? Are you sure? Moscow *blat* usually cost more.'

Vitaly had a doping control to perform the next day. He went to Igor Zagorskiy at work and told him the entire story. Zagorskiy took the 10,000 roubles and swapped them for the magic document that would save him from the draft.

Vitaly skipped to the travel office in Rossport. The woman at the desk frowned.

'A new passport? Do you want to wait and wait and wait like an ordinary citizen?'

Vitaly understood. He put 30,000 roubles into another envelope and handed it over with his application. A fresh passport appeared within days. Vitaly's faith in the system was restored entirely.

And so, through the deep quirks of Russian life, it came to pass that the celebrated hammer thrower Tatyana Lysenko didn't go to the Beijing Olympics. But Vitaly Stepanov did. He worked on WADA's Outreach programme, putting athletes and coaches in contact with the anti-doping world.

Exhibit E

Vitaly and another DCO went to an amateur sailing champion-ship on a lake outside Moscow. They needed to come back with thirty-five samples. The first problem was that there were only thirty-two competitors. They were all hobbyists. The well-to-do class of the oligarch era, sailing their boats and boasting about whose sloop was biggest.

The sailors returned to shore. Vitaly implored people to pro-vide samples. The absence of any chaperones was a loophole that meant that even a sample containing enough chemicals to con-taminate a lake would get a free pass. Numbers were numbers, though. Some sailors laughed when asked to pee into the pots.

'I am walking from my big yacht to my big car. That tells you enough about me. You are a prospector and courier of urine. That tells me enough about you. I will keep walking. Have a nice day.'

'I'm sorry but we're from Rusada.'

'I don't care if you are from the Kremlin. This is my hobby. If you want to disqualify me then please do.'

Somehow, Vitaly and his colleague ended up with twenty samples. Completely pointless, but Rusada could invoice for twenty fees.

Sometimes you have to just go along to get along.

Chapter 8

No one could accuse Vitaly and Yuliya of hanging around. Everything was on fast forward and Vitaly was entranced and at times bewildered. After two and a half dates he was still unsure if this girl even liked him. Then Yuliya suggested that he might visit Kursk with her.

'Kursk?' he said. 'Really? Why?'

'To meet my family.'

Already? he thought to himself. *I've only known her two weeks.* It wouldn't be plain sailing. He was reticent in company and a non-drinker. Her family weren't guaranteed to like him.

In Kursk, to escape family scrutiny they went running together. Not far from where she lived there was a route Yuliya liked, and if you could avoid being attacked by the mean and mangy dogs that wandered about and the old woman who screamed vitriol at passers-by, it was an okay sort of run.

When they were done running they did strides on a disused soccer pitch. While striding they talked about marriage, just in a general sense. It was a light-hearted conversation – the pluses, the minuses and the abstractions. And then Vitaly steered the conversation back to the two of them.

'We could get married.'

'Yeah, yeah, yeah!'

Vitaly was laughing, Yuliya too. It was a joke, right?

Right.

Vitaly then dropped to one knee. His question had waited long enough.

'Will you marry me, please?'

If you like you romance served in syrup of clichés there was nothing romantic about this. No sunset, no flowers. They'd known each other for two weeks and he didn't have a ring.

'Yes, of course I will marry you.'

This conversation was a joke, wasn't it? Vitaly more or less agreed with her.

'Yes. A joke. Why, what did you think?'

Except that a seed had been planted. And the next day it flowered.

'I am serious about marriage.'

'Okay,' she replied.

He took that as a yes.

That weekend in Kursk there was no celebration. When Yuliya told her mum that she and Vitaly were going to get married, Lyubov cried. They were not tears of joy.

'You've known him two weeks. This is crazy.'

She'd already asked her mum and her sisters what they thought of Vitaly. 'He doesn't drink. He doesn't speak and he's seems grumpy.'

'Apart from that . . . anything?'

How could Yuliya begin to explain?

Things had happened in the past that had changed her outlook. Her father's drinking had caused nightmares and often brought horror to the daylight hours. She recalled one evening when she was at home alone, hoping he wouldn't come home drunk but knowing he would. By then Lyubov had taken steps to lessen the violence. The apartment was hers, not his, and so if he didn't come straight from work the apartment door would be locked and he would be refused entry.

Three hours after work, a knock. Yuliya silently stole to the door and saw him through the peephole. He was drunk. She tiptoed back into the kitchen and sat on the floor. The knocking got louder but she dared not budge.

'I know you're in there,' he shouted. 'Open the door.'

He began to bang more aggressively. She sobbed, knowing this wouldn't end well. He shouted, swore, promised violence on whoever was inside. She was sure he would break the door down. Then his frustration, anger, self-loathing would rain down on her head. For some time, she had truly believed that he would kill someone. Most likely Lyubov, but maybe even one of them, his daughters. Yuliya was more defiant than Katia and Gelia but she too was scared. On the kitchen floor, now she cried as the thumping grew more furious and she braced for the splintering noise of the door crashing open. At that moment she prayed.

Finally, the noise stopped and he left, probably to his mother's apartment. Grandma Alla wouldn't turn him away. She too had suffered beatings, though, and sometimes she would leave him in her apartment, preferring to sleep rough in the park, under the stars, than wait for his next attack.

Yuliya could see no excuses for him. It wasn't that he didn't know the way alcohol affected him. A week of drinking would be followed by a week of recovery. A never-ending cycle of misery. During his recovery week he still needed an occasional drink to steady things. And it wasn't that Igor didn't understand the implications of his addiction. Once, he had agreed to go a local hospital to have an Antabuse implant fitted that would block the breakdown of alcohol and cause extreme sickness within minutes of taking any. The medication would be effective for up to twelve months.

With the implant, Igor didn't drink for eight months. One evening he decided to go to Tutova, the tiny village where

Lyubov's parents lived. He asked Yuliya to accompany him. That night she dreamed he would resume drinking in Tutova. After they got there, he went out to meet a friend and it was inevitable. Yuliya lit the open fire. And waited. Back he came, drunk and with a bottle of vodka. He took a drink from the bottle and vomited violently. Then he took another drink and got sick again. He kept doing this until the vodka was gone. Drink. Vomit. Drink. After that he persuaded Lyubov to take him back to the hospital. The implant was removed. After that, a week-long descent into alcohol-induced mayhem became a three-week binge.

Yuliya recalled another day, when Igor was with the family in their apartment. He was relatively sober but agitated. Then suddenly he was on the balcony, spraying one of the girls' perfumes into a small glass. Lyubov took the perfume from his hand as he sucked the last drops from the glass.

How to explain the seductiveness of security?

It haunted Yuliya that Grandpa Mikhail had been the unlucky one. Her grandparents were the two people who she knew truly loved her. Igor had claimed he hadn't killed his father-in-law. No one had believed him. And no one wanted to testify against him. Except Yuliya.

'Everyone was afraid,' she told Vitaly. 'My sisters, our neighbours, they thought what happens when he gets out of prison? He will remember who spoke against him. I didn't care. I wanted to say he was a very violent person when he drank.'

Up to the day before Igor's trial began, Yuliya was testifying against her father. Whether by deliberate omission or otherwise, nobody had given notice to the court that Yuliya was to be a witness. Her words were never heard. As things turned out, they hadn't been necessary. Her father was handed his seven years. Seldom was a sentence pronounced that brought such relief to the family of the accused.

After Igor went to prison, a lawyer had come to the apartment. He said that he could arrange for the prison term to be shortened. It would cost money, but it could be done. They told him they weren't interested. Yuliya remembers the startled expression in the man's eyes. He couldn't fathom it. Her only thought was that if she could pay money to make the sentence longer, she would do it. The lawyer's journey was wasted.

The infection that would bring Yuliya down with tuberculosis had waited for the right moment. It arrived not long after her father's trial, when Yuliya still felt drained and weak. Regardless of her diet of supplements and vitamins, in early 2006 she became very sick with the old-fashioned ailment, a condition that now haunted Russia again after the breakdown of the old Soviet health services. Yuliya was coughing, feeling fatigued and lacking in appetite and by March she had been diagnosed with TB.

If she responded to a bombardment of antibiotics she would recover, yet the onset of TB was treated like a little death. With the usual Russian despondency, her friends told her solemnly that she would never run again. There would be no escape now. Kursk had won. The city had invaded her lungs and laid siege to her. The Russian medical system is a lottery with not a lot of grand prizes. But there is a bias that favours the young. Get sick at a tender age and you have a better chance. Luckily Yuliya was young. She had a doctor assigned to her in the hospital who was a very good man and very enlightened. He promised her that it would take time but that she would race again. She believed him. She would be fine.

During her three months in the hospital, her boyfriend at the time never showed up once. Unlike Vladimir Mokhnev, her coach, who haunted the place. He came to visit every second day, often bringing fruit, endearing himself to a young woman who had lost a grandfather she loved and whose father had just been sent to prison.

Like most Russian children, physical education classes had been a part of her daily school life. A kid had to achieve certain marks in running just to graduate to the next year's grade. Yuliya had always loved the PE classes and usually performed better than most of her classmates in her running tests. She was just faster. She was faster than most of the boys. She was sure she had some talent. When she was eleven a teacher had brought her to a cross-city event in Kursk and had she not won a medal? Her first time in a proper competition. She'd made Grandpa Mikhail smile. He told her that she could really be something, anything. This little flea of a girl who could fly. And then? Nothing. She was thirteen before another teacher brought her to another event, and this time, to her surprise, she didn't win. Then she was fourteen and it was all over. She was washed up.

Finally, when she was sixteen and in college, another teacher asked her to make up the numbers in a competition. She ran for the college in a city 500 metres event and came third. Only the winner got a medal. Yuliya got a certificate. You never saw anybody on a podium at the Olympics kissing a certificate, but she was encouraged. So she decided that for the event next year she would train herself properly and she would come back with a medal to show everybody. She would make sure that the only shiny object being handed out at her next event went home in her pocket.

She began to train seriously in the summer of 2003. After four months or so, the race came around again. All the best kids in the city gathered up to race. And Yuliya. This time she figured that she was ready, though. To her disgust, she came second to Kristina Khaleeva, who would eventually become a friend but who that day seemed like the spawn of the devil. It was explained to Yuliya that Khaleeva had been training for far longer than a few months. This was Khaleeva's life, not her little hobby.

But Yuliya had shown enough potential. She had earned the right to make it her life too. Her teacher was impressed enough to point her in the direction of a coach who could help her improve. 'The best coach in Kursk,' he said, like that was some big deal. So she went to see this coach. His name was Vladimir Mokhnev. He seemed like he was a big deal, acted that way.

She enjoyed training. She liked Mokhnev. She was making new friends and doing well, and the need to train gave her an excuse not to be at home. She was hungrier than the other kids, eyeing them wolfishly. Who was here just for the fun? Who had some edge? Would any of them kill for the chance to make a living from running? She would. Not literally but almost.

She got faster and faster. Top three in the city. Top three in the region. She started travelling to national competitions for her age group. She didn't always win medals but sometimes she got out of Kursk, which showed she was going places. She saw new towns and cities and she ran in them. And she understood that the girls who were running faster than her and who were beating her to medals had all trained for years more than she had. They were honed. In their cities and villages, they were the ones who would do what was needed to satisfy their hunger. But she would catch them.

In Kursk the girls down at training had other explanations.

'They are beating you, Yuliya, because of what they take, not what they do.'

Huh?

'Yeah, yeah, they have been training for years. Yeah, they have big-shot coaches and better running gear than you have. But those big-shot coaches give them pills to make them run faster. Wise up. It's not just hunger. It's pills and injections and hunger. When you have trained for as long as they have, when you are skinny and your stomach is a hard skillet, they will still be faster because of what they pop into their mouths with a glass of water and into their arms with a needle. Wake up and smell the Dianabol, Yuliya.'

She had asked Mokhnev about these magic beans and he had brushed her off. 'Too soon. Not now.' And she had doubted him. Doubted if he was all that he made himself out to be.

Now, he arrived reliably with his fruit and his smile, and duly she fell for his kindness. And as things developed between them, she believed him when he said he would leave his wife for her. Early on Yuliya had discussed the situation with Lyubov.

'I am thinking of cheating on my boyfriend.'

'Why?'

'Because I have met someone else. Did you ever cheat on my father?'

'What do you think? He was drunk a lot of the time. He beat me. He paid no attention to me.'

Lyubov told Yuliya that when they lived at the nature reserve she'd had a lover. He was good with his hands and he had made her a wardrobe. One day Igor had worked out what was going on and, returning home, he hauled the wardrobe from their bedroom, dragged it outside, smashed it with an axe and set fire to it. No words necessary. Lyubov was telling her daughter, take your happiness where you can find it.

Yuliya liked Mokhnev. He wasn't a good man but neither was he the worst man she had known. She knew plenty about bad men. She was the seed of a bad man. She had been magnetically drawn to bad men no matter how bad they were to her. She was young still and not undamaged. She dreamed pragmatic dreams. Survival stuff, not fair princesses in castles with towers and knights on white steeds. Those dreams were for other girls. Yuliya's mind performed the maths of survival. The geometry of getting through, getting out, getting on. Men wanted sex usually and mainly. That was a simple equation. Deal with it and keep your eye on the dream. And, as Lyubov said, take your happiness wherever you find it.

And so it had begun. The intimacy, the complicity, their shared savage hunger that, they hoped, would get them to Moscow and beyond.

Chapter 9

September 2009, offices of Rusada
Another conversation between Vitaly and Director Sinev

'Come in, Vitaly.'

'I won't keep you long.'

'Well, I'm here one way or the other till you drive me home this evening, so don't worry about that. Keep me for as long as you like. What's up?'

'You know that girl I told you about?'

'The runner. You are going to Sochi with her, of course, of course.'

'Well, there's more. I am going to marry her on 10 October.'

'On 10 October? Next month? In a few weeks?'

'Yes. In Kursk.'

'In Kursk? Well . . .'

'If you could come, I would really like that.'

'Kursk. On 10 October. A wedding? Your wedding? You do work fast. That is a sprint, Vitaly. But congratulations, my friend. I am happy for you.'

'Thank you, Director Sinev, and again I would really like it if you could come.'

Vitaly's parents didn't know that their son was harbouring a girlfriend in Moscow. Vitaly couldn't be entirely sure of it himself. Yuliya was like a feral cat. Not to be owned. She was to be fed and amused. So when he called his parents to say that he would be getting married imminently, he sensed a shiver of déjà vu. This wasn't the first time he had announced a dramatic twist in his life.

'So we would love for you to be in Kursk for our wedding,' he said.

'We will try to be there,' his parents said. 'What's her name again?'

'Yuliya. Oh, and one other thing. There will be no alcohol at the wedding.'

Once, when he was a child, Vitaly had seen his father drunk. Sergey was a silly and infrequent drunk and Vitaly hadn't liked that edition of his dad. The foolishness didn't amuse him, the disappearance of dignity was disappointing. And the more he saw of alcohol's hold on Russian life, the less he liked it. Surely to celebrate a happy occasion like a wedding, people could eat, laugh and dance. Not that he was overly keen on dancing. If people were happy, though, why did they need to drink? Why did Russian celebrations need to be fuelled by vodka?

'In Russia we need to have alcohol,' his father demurred. 'That is tradition. That is culture. That is how we honour guests. She's not Amish, is she?'

'No, Dad. Yuliya and her family would prefer alcohol,' Vitaly said. 'But this is my wedding, too. We will honour them with food and a party. Can they not honour us by not drinking for one evening? If they are happy for us, do they have to drink as well?'

'Thanks for explaining,' said his father as if he had been missing a key point.

Yuliya's family were also bewildered. No alcohol equalled no guests.

'If there is no vodka nobody will come.'

'They will come to celebrate with us.'

'They won't. They celebrate with vodka.'

It stood that way until mid–September, when Vitaly was in Sochi with Yuliya and the deadlock broke. He learned that in Kursk a marathon originally scheduled for 3 October had been postponed for a week until 10 October. The day of his wedding. A lightbulb flickered. He went to Yuliya.

'I have an idea for you and your family. I will accept a wedding with alcohol if you let me run the marathon on the morning of the wedding.'

She stared at him blankly. What fresh lunacy now?

He explained how in the spring he'd run himself to exhaustion in the Moscow marathon. The experience had wasted him and elated him. He had found another depth in himself. A few weekends later he had been staying at his Aunt Anna's apartment in Moscow, helping with his little cousin, Stepan. On the Saturday morning they'd driven to a 10k race to give Vitaly his running fix for the weekend. That evening he read there was a marathon being held the following morning near Nizhny Novgorod, just a five-hour drive from Moscow. It was late but, like a man possessed, he gathered his gear and said farewell to his baffled aunt. He was going out. He might be some time.

He was on the road by midnight. He was over the speed limit within minutes. The inevitable. *Gaishniki*. Traffic cops. A routine shakedown.

'You were really speeding,' the officer said.

'I have to get to a marathon,' Vitaly said. An unimpeachable justification as if it were a medical emergency he alone was qualified to deal with.

'Well, 5,000 roubles should get you to the starting line.'

Vitaly had 3,000 roubles in his pocket. He needed fuel and petrol. Food would be good too.

They haggled. And haggled more. Finally, the cop did his maths. He could have trousered four soft shakedowns in the time he was losing with this stringy fanatic. He accepted 1,000 roubles with bad grace.

At 8 a.m. Vitaly pulled in near the starting line. He had one hour in which to steal some sleep if his brain switched off. It didn't.

The course was cast out in a loop, 13 miles out, 13 back. It was a hot morning. He ran the first half like an athlete but hobbled homewards like a wounded soldier searching for his regiment. Then he collapsed into his car. He had been awake for thirty straight hours, very few of which had been sedentary. Now he had to drive back to join the Sunday-evening traffic in Moscow so that early in the morning he could collect Director Sinev and drive him to work.

He told Yuliya all this so that the idea of running a marathon on the morning of his wedding to her might seem reasonable. Wearily she nodded.

'Whatever makes you happy, Vitaly.'

It would be his most successful negotiation with Yuliya for quite some time.

The Stepanovs met their daughter-in-law-to-be on the day before the wedding. Neither family was religious but Kursk has many churches and cathedrals and inevitably they ended up in somebody else's place of worship. They visited the Original Kursk Root Spring Church, where there were spring pools of sacred water and a glinting river. It was a serene, moonlit evening and the Stepanovs allowed themselves the thought that perhaps Vitaly wasn't entirely mad after all.

The next morning, while Yuliya dressed to be wed, Vitaly ran around Kursk for two hours and forty-one minutes. His best time yet for a marathon. He wondered if the distance had been a little short of regulation but he took it all to be a happy omen. He told himself this marriage would be another marathon. Some easy parts and more hard parts but he would keep going.

They signed the papers at the registry office and had the reception in a restaurant. Fifty or so people. Some drinks. No fights.

Vitaly was quiet and declined to either drink or dance. Yuliya's family was generously populated with big drinkers and clodding dancers, and Vitaly was an odd addition to their world. Yuliya spent no time explaining him to her people. Vitaly was fit for purpose. Anything else wasn't her problem. She knew that he loved her. Maybe someday she would love him. If not? For now, he was fit for purpose.

Unofficially the bosses in Rusada gave Vitaly and Yuliya a nine-day honeymoon trip to Egypt. They travelled to Israel as well. They saw the holy sites and the Dead Sea. They had conversations about doping and Yuliya's preparations. Nothing changed. No conversions. They never got near the road to Damascus.

When they returned home Yuliya packed a bag for training camp. Business as usual. Vitaly prepared to go back to his own job but the fundamental problem still grew in his mind. He was returning to Rusada to do his anti-doping work. He was kissing his wife goodbye as she headed off to her job as a fully doped athlete. He raised the issue one more time before she left.

'Do you think you should change the way that you prepare?'

'I have to prepare the way I always have prepared. I have told you that.'

'But maybe you should try something different.'

'Maybe, seeing as how you don't really know anything, you should just not say anything.'

Conversation over, she left. *That thing people say*, thought Vitaly, *about the honeymoon being over? I get that.*

He glanced toward a forlorn pile in the corner of the flat. The photos and film of their wedding had arrived. They sat unopened. Neither the groom nor the bridegroom had bothered with them.

Chapter 10

They hadn't been married long. Since the honeymoon they'd had just the odd weekend in each other's company, which he sensed Yuliya was fine with. They fought a lot when they were apart. Text conversations ended in conflict, phone calls ended suddenly and without goodbyes. He was due some time off towards the end of the year and so thought he would go to a training camp at Belgorod, 700 kilometres from Moscow, in December to be with her. Maybe time together would help. When he told her his plan to come to Belgorod, though, he felt her lack of enthusiasm. If there was any joy, she concealed it.

He phoned her on the way to Belgorod. He was making good time, he said, and hoped to arrive late this evening instead of tomorrow morning. Yuliya responded as if she wasn't bothered either way. If anything it might be better if he arrived tomorrow. It wasn't her idea for him to come. He could stay in Kursk for the night and drive on the next morning. It really didn't matter to her.

'Yuliya, we are family now,' he said, discouraged. 'We should be together as much as possible.'

'Not again, Vitaly. I am a runner. I want to compete well. If you don't like that, that's your problem.'

Vitaly would tell himself to keep going. This might feel like a steeplechase but really it was a marathon.

After Belgorod they spent the rest of December in Kursk and

then stayed on through the traditional Russian holiday period of early January. Vitaly was uncomfortable in Kursk. He had no rapport with Yuliya's sisters or mother. They found him odd. The shadow of Igor's life and death hung over them still. As for Yuliya, they hoped for her sake that running could take her out of Kursk. This made it hard for them to warm to Mr Doping Control and his puritanical attitude to alcohol. Eventually Vitaly and Yuliya returned to Moscow. The change hadn't been as good as a rest. Neither was the return.

Early in 2010, Rusada had good news for Vitaly. WADA wanted him to work on their Outreach programme at the Vancouver Winter Olympics beginning on 10 February. Maybe they saw him as a poster boy for their cause: if a Russian can be committed, then shouldn't we all be? Vitaly was pleased but not as excited as he'd been two years before when departing for the Summer Games in Beijing. Back then he'd seen himself as part of a new generation changing sport. Now he knew a lot more and believed a lot less. He was the anti-doping crusader whose wife used her banned drugs in front of him. Her casual insouciance felt like the insult on top of the injury. When Yuliya referred to doping, it was only to remind him how the 'real world' worked.

Twice in the weeks since the honeymoon they had set out for the registry office, resigned to ending a marriage that wasn't working. In Russia if a couple has no children and no property then divorce is a simple administrative matter. The unhappy couple present at the registry office. Both sign a form.

I, Vitaly, want to divorce Yuliya.

I, Yuliya, want to divorce Vitaly.

We have no children and we have no property.

If one or both returns and signs the form again one month later then the couple are divorced. Both passports are then stamped to indicate the change of marital status. In a country that otherwise values bureaucracy, it is the simplest of processes. A simple process that didn't work out for Yuliya and Vitaly.

The first time, they were on their way but somehow talked each other out of divorce while stuck in traffic before heading home in fraught silence. The second time, they made it to the registry office but found it closed for a state holiday. Vitaly felt weighed down by it all. Still married but only because of chance.

~

Though he wasn't in the mood for fireworks, Vitaly attended Vancouver's opening ceremony. With his WADA accreditation he was able to take an 'Olympic family' shuttle from the hotel, sitting beside an elderly gentleman from the International Olympic Committee (IOC). The man was seventyish, Vitaly reckoned. Middle-aged in IOC terms. Close to the stadium the traffic slowed and was then halted by protestors. With the engine switched off and no air circulating, the shuttle suddenly felt suffocating. An even older man than Vitaly's neighbour became distressed and short of breath. People were panicking.

'You have to let him out. You have to let other people out too. We aren't moving. It is too hot. Do something!'

The man continued to gasp for air.

The driver was in an impossible position. Inside the shuttle bus the air was hot and stifling, but nobody could be allowed off the bus. So that they could be whisked straight to the VIP zone inside the security loop, the 'Olympic family' passengers had cleared security back at their luxury hotel. While they were on the bus they were in the loop. If they left the bus here, they would be out of the loop. They were trapped within their own VIP cordon sanitaire.

The old man was in serious trouble. Finally, two volunteers arrived and took him away. The rest of the passengers were bustled through to the VIP zone. There to recount stories of how they had come face to face with strange people not much in love with the Olympics. Something Vitaly's neighbour said would stay with him: that the biggest problem with the International Olympic Committee was too many old people.

For Vitaly, Vancouver was just work. No joy. His innocence had made Beijing a dream. In Vancouver in his free time he ran instead of watching sport. Most of what he saw of the Winter Olympics he watched on the television above his treadmill. Stacy Spletzer noticed the change. This wasn't the bright, happy young man she recalled from Beijing.

'What has happened to you, Vitaly?'

He told her that plenty had happened. He used to believe that Russia was on the point of changing. Now he knew it wasn't. Doping was more institutionalised than he had ever imagined. The stories he'd told them in Beijing about the early doping control trips? Athletes who were present but not available for testing, and coaches who believed they could nominate who should be tested, all that was just the tip of the iceberg. What lay beneath was the real problem.

Oh, and something else. He'd got himself married.

Spletzer sensed that Vitaly needed more than just a chatty catch-up. She asked if there was anything specific that he would like done. He said he wanted to talk to somebody. Somebody high up within WADA. He would like that person to be Stuart Kemp.

'We'll make that happen,' she said.

Two days later, Vitaly sat with Kemp and Spletzer at a quiet table in the cafe in the athletes' village and told his story.

'Rusada is a joke,' he said. 'We paint stripes on a donkey and pretend it's a zebra.'

Spletzer and Kemp exchanged glances. This was way above their pay grade.

Days later, Vitaly came to a private gathering in a room within the official WADA hotel. A small group sat waiting for him. The meeting was secret and the arrangements cloak-and-dagger. Vitaly asked if the meeting room would destroy itself when they left. Nervous smiles.

Stuart Kemp was present as the link man. There was an American there called Richard Young, whose name didn't register with Vitaly but who told a story about figure skaters and doping that suggested he worked in or with laboratories. A suave Norwegian called Rune Andersen told Vitaly that just yesterday he'd met with Vitaly Mutko, the Russian Minister of Sports, who had boasted everything back home was good.[1]

'So, Vitaly,' Rune Andersen said, 'how are we going to fight this?'

'That's what I came to ask you.'

Andersen didn't stay long and, after he left, Vitaly recounted everything he knew. The doping control missions, the official indifference. Rusada's habit of only looking in places where it would find nothing.

'If we stumble across a positive it can be disappeared for a small fee,' Vitaly said, 'but we only stumble over them. Nothing is targeted. We are in the business of showing that we did many tests and we deliver plenty of positives, but those who test positive are carefully chosen from the second or third tier. They show that Russian sport is clean. People look at the numbers and mistakenly believe we are serious about doping. Nobody asks who you were testing and when and for what. We just show the numbers and keep the business going.'

He tried to convey how the singular harshness of his nation's history might be inextricable from its approach to sport. Athletes in other countries might see athletics as a way of adding to their lives; many Russian athletes saw it as the only way to a life. For an athlete it was an escape. For the state it was propaganda.

A country that had been hermetically sealed for so long now wanted to show it was strong and powerful.

One of the WADA people asked if Vitaly felt he had any allies within the organisation. Superficially it seemed to be a reasonable question. Nobody in the room found it odd. This was Rusada, the agency created to police Russian sport, which had been nurtured under WADA's wing. And the question was really whether or not, in the fight against doping, Vitaly had any support at all inside the anti-doping body of Mother Russia.

Vitaly had asked himself this many times before. He mentioned a couple of names but said he couldn't be sure of them. There was another guy, Sergey Pervakov, who might be useful. Then he paused before offering another name, someone he wasn't sure about but who could be very useful.

'Maybe Oleg Samsonov,' he said.

Samsonov. In the bear pit of online chat rooms he had been a dissonant presence. Particularly in the online forum of the newspaper *Sport Express*. Prowling, lupine and equipped with a wealth of information about Russian sport, Samsonov used his knowledge like incisors, tearing opponents apart. His sharp teeth made him unassailable in an argument. Trolls and cranks feared him. His contributions were written under a pseudonym but noticed nevertheless. People at Rusada read the posts and knew they were written by a man connected to someone on the inside. The fingerprints suggested the author was the shambling Oleg Samsonov. He was not long in the employ of Rusada. Aleksandr Derevoedov, the head of the medical department, also believed to be a pseudonymous frequenter of the same forum, had offered him the chance to come and work for the organisation. Flattered that his expertise had been noted, Samsonov had accepted. He was a mildly derelict figure, almost fifty and with a weariness that made him interesting. His pallor suggested a bad diet and long nights before the dim glow of a computer screen. He gave the impression that daylight and fresh air weren't the sort of things he was looking for in life.

Vitaly soon found Samsonov a useful ally when talking to the bosses about strategy and targeted testing. Most staffers were content to run up the numbers in return for a wage, but Samsonov grasped the bigger picture. Anybody with brains could see the big picture, but Samsonov was willing to deal with what he saw.

They had travelled together by car on the weekend of the Outreach programme that had brought Yuliya into Vitaly's orbit. Samsonov made a good companion for Director Sinev, who had been tagging along. Both were diabetic. Every time they stopped for food, Vitaly nagged them with an almost paternal fondness. 'Eat sensibly, men. You know what happens if you don't.' They'd groaned in harmony and told him to mind his own business, but still heeded him. There was a lot about Samsonov that weekend that Vitaly had liked.

'For Health and Fairness in Sport' was Outreach's slogan and they'd made up their minds about people depending upon whether or not they dropped by the booth. Yuliya included. Valentin Maslakov, a former sprinter and now head coach of the national team, had declined to come to the booth.[2] Vitaly asked him several times and each time he had refused. The antidote to Maslakov was Russian 800 metres hero Yuriy Borzakovskiy. The great champion called by the booth and Vitaly fondly recalled his famous gold–medal victory at the 2004 Athens Games.

None of these musings were what WADA wanted to hear, however.

Samsonov had helped Vitaly see the pattern. Not long after he had first ambled into the Rusada office, Samsonov saw what Vitaly was getting at and how the system was being corrupted. They decided that if they could plan the missions and decide who should be tested, it would be a start.

This was more like what Vitaly's WADA audience had gathered for.

'So, were you able to change things?'

Vitaly shook his head. No, they had hit a dead end. The bosses didn't want them concerning themselves with such matters. Management decreed who should be tested and when. If the rationale was unclear to all colleagues, well, it wasn't necessary for everything to be clearly understood. He and Samsonov had tried to show them there was a better way. The bosses duly conceded that, yes, that might be the case and they were pleased to have their input, but they were the bosses and they had decided.

Samsonov was head of the Results Management Department, an important job. He had been hired on the basis of his broad understanding of these matters. He and Vitaly sometimes wondered if, by employing him, the bosses had merely wished to silence Oleg Samsonov's online voice. At first, Samsonov seemed philosophical both about being neutered and about the failure to convince the bosses, but as time passed Vitaly noticed a change in him. Samsonov stopped fighting the battles and making the arguments. His mind was on something else. Vitaly couldn't say what but he watched and wondered.

Samsonov passed a lot of time chatting with athletes. Vitaly couldn't help overhearing snippets of conversation, and not all of Samsonov's enquiries were connected to his immediate duties. Vitaly reckoned he was trawling for information, finding out things that mapped the terrain for him. It seemed that Samsonov had gained many athletes' confidence. To Vitaly it didn't seem quite right but, having himself married a doped athlete, he didn't feel he could really make an ethical issue out of it. On the other hand, he could see that in being cosy with athletes, Samsonov was leaving himself open to whispering campaigns. Russians whispers can be malignant.

'Something else,' Vitaly said to his WADA audience. 'Samsonov had a black notebook.'

They leaned forward. More attentive now. A notebook?

In the notebook were recorded all the sample numbers that either the Ministry or the Moscow anti-doping laboratory had asked about. There was a pattern. A telephone call from the Ministry or the lab. Always the same routine: they had only a sample number and could we please tell them who it belongs to? Decisions would then be made – positive or negative? Director Sinev knew it wasn't right and got Samsonov to make a record of every request. He kept the details in a notebook in his office at Rusada.

'We'd be really interested in seeing this notebook,' said one of the WADA people.

'Actually, that's a problem now,' Vitaly said.

'How so?'

'Oleg Samsonov is in prison.'

In the end they thanked him. They knew he was well intentioned but they weren't sure everything he said was to be believed. Even if it was, what could they do? Their own WADA code had been framed to preclude them from formally investigating a country. Sport in Russia was meant to be policed by Rusada. WADA's hands were bound with their own silk. No one at WADA had ever imagined an entire national agency turning rogue. Rusada could say their donkey was a zebra but WADA couldn't come and check this out to its own satisfaction.

When they were done and all hands had been shaken again, Vitaly thought of Yuliya and her advice to him about finding out how the real world worked. Perhaps this was it. He noticed, in the real world of this hotel room with the anti-drugs czars, that everybody had seemed to studiously ignore the fact that Vitaly had told them from the outset that his wife was doping. In fact, in conversation they'd ignored her existence entirely.

Nobody had asked Vitaly what his wife's name was. Or if they were happy together.

Welcome to the real world.

The next day, Stacy arranged for Vitaly to go to Whistler Mountain for three days to be part of the educational team running the other Outreach booth there. In Whistler he enjoyed his running a little more. The still, cold air and the majestic views mended him a little. He passed road signs warning of bears crossing. He was Russian and he had never seen a bear. He had come to the Winter Olympics and the thing he most wanted to see was a bear.

He had promised the WADA people that while he was in Whistler he would write to them with suggestions. No solutions came to him, though. He needed WADA to tell him what to do, not the other way around. He wrote a short note, telling them that if he learned anything else he'd let them know. Their response was one he would hear many times.

'Thanks. Be careful. Stay safe.'

He brought his low mood home with him. When Mr Derevoedov and Director Sinev asked for a report in the style of his breathless Beijing summary, he wrote one line: 'I was doing Outreach for WADA. And when I wasn't, I was at my hotel.'

Chapter 11

Moscow was cold. Vitaly found no warmth either at home or at work.

His downbeat mood added to the disenchantment between him and his employers. Director Sinev, Mr Derevoedov and Natalia Govorkova, the financial director – and even Zagorskiy, whom he viewed as an equal – would stop at his desk and engage in brief conversations. They all sensed his disillusion and he picked up on their disappointment in him. Even Sinev's conviviality had dried up.

Vitaly had worked hard and efficiently. Nobody could argue with that, but they couldn't hide misgivings about his attitude, his approach to the job. His lack of understanding of unique but traditional Russian values was a problem. It was all a little unpatriotic. They seemed jaded by the stream of complaints from federations who were sore because Vitaly was so inflexible. They thought he was pretty high and mighty for somebody who married an athlete no different from any other Russian athlete.

From the Rusada offices he trudged through the snow and wondered which he would lose first – his job or his wife.

In Vancouver he had been out of sight and out of mind. Soon after he got back, it was the weekend of the National Indoor Championships, which were being held in Moscow. Yuliya had dreamed of little else while he was away.

Yuliya had asked her friend Zina to come from Kursk for the

championships. He recalled Zina from the wedding. She had made a lovely gesture. Vitaly wasn't drinking alcohol so she proposed a toast asking everybody to drink just orange juice. But, considering how little he saw of Yuliya these days, did she really need to summon a friend for the one weekend she would be with him in Moscow? He would just have to roll with it, he told himself.

He sat alone in the stands and brooded until Sergey Pervakov, his colleague from Rusada, came along. Pervakov was one of the few colleagues who took an interest in the big picture. At the meeting in Vancouver, Vitaly had mentioned him as a possible ally. Pervakov had come to Rusada to train as a doping control officer and had become good at the job. He was straight and firm and Vitaly had been able to wangle him a promotion. Pervakov was now helping out in the planning department.

Vitaly neither liked nor trusted Natalia Vaganova, the head of planning. She had worked for Rossport and came to Rusada to help Russia win medals, whatever it took. For Vaganova, planning was a simple equation. Hit the target number of tests with the minimum amount of damage. Keep the communication lines between athletes and labs open.

She probably would have brought a colleague from Rossport into the planning department, but Vitaly still had some influence with Director Sinev. With Oleg Samsonov, he had gone to Sinev several times about the planning situation. They could do a much better job than Vaganova and, though Sinev could see what they meant, he shook his head. No. As Director he knew removing the head of planning was too much, too radical. Planning was the key to the preparation of the country's best athletes. Meddling there would be like signing the death warrant for his career. Pervakov's transfer had been a sop. Vitaly hoped Pervakov would be his man on the inside of the planning department.

That evening in Moscow, Yuliya failed to make the 800 metres indoor final. Vitaly could immediately see the gathering storm in her eyes. She had come to win. He felt as if he was trespassing on her privacy when he offered his words of thin comfort.

He was torn by his ambivalence. Did he want her doping programme to be a success? Did he want to travel on those coat-tails? On the other hand, he was enjoying the fruits of his wife being a well-rewarded elite athlete and the main contributor to the family income. A voice inside his head reminded him that he hadn't asked her to hand back any of her prize money. Another voice smirked about him being the anti-doping officer who had knowingly married a doping athlete. Had he seriously addressed that little contradiction? If winning makes her happy and doping makes her win, what's your position then? He was the man who spent his working day trying to expose doping athletes and yet he was married to a woman who doped.

Seeing her fail to reach the National Indoor 800 metres final brought out the runner in him. He felt for her and tried to be supportive. But she could see through the platitudes and on a night like this she resented what he stood for. Mr Fucking Anti-Doping. So she picked the fight that he wanted to avoid. She told him she would rather be doped to the gills than be as bang full of shit as he was.

'Let me know when you arrive in the real world, Vitaly. Then you can try to say these stupid things you are thinking.'

'But—'

'Are you my coach? No. You are not my coach. I don't even know what the fuck you are doing here.'

'I'm your husband.'

'Are you my coach?'

'No.'

'Exactly. Go away.'

Back in the stands, Pervakov had something to tell Vitaly. He had been working on the test planning for the National Championships, the logistics of who would be tested and where. That was the theory anyway. He leaned in close to Vitaly. Rusada, he said, hadn't planned any of it. Alexei Melnikov had arranged everything that needed to be done.[1] Who would be tested, for what and when. These decisions were handed down to Rusada by the national head coach. Pervakov had come to understand that the planning department was part of the system that supported doping in Russia. In other words, his own bosses at Rusada were protecting the things he had hoped to fight when he first turned up for work at the national anti-doping agency.

Vitaly thought about the journey back from the CSKA stadium and reckoned it would be better for him to leave early and make his own way home to the apartment. But he couldn't do that because each race was to him like a short story that he had to finish.

What Pervakov told him had added another important piece to the jigsaw and confirmed what Yuliya had said on the night of their first date: Rusada exists to help the athletes cheat. *Yeah*, Vitaly thought, *but only those whom the system deems worth protecting.* How many of the competitors in front of him were within the magic circle of state-approved doping? How many others were hoping to get into the protected group? Talent was appreciated but it didn't win medals, at least not on its own.

Was there anybody down there who knew what the system offered and said thanks, but no thanks? Who preferred to be an honest also-ran? Probably not. You wanted to escape your grim city, make a life for yourself and those you loved. So you put your heart and soul into running. The culture didn't stigmatise cheating. The culture said it was the smart thing to do. You say you want to do something for yourself and for your family? But you won't do this? You'll live in this dirt and shit and make everybody else do the same because you have some notion about a purity that has never existed. Good luck with that. Who would have the strength to say thanks but no thanks?

Doping was just another Russian way of going along to get along. The system wasn't comfortable with the presence of dissidents, especially those claiming the moral high ground. Vitaly suspected everybody he was watching was doped and that in a perverse way they were all starting from the same point. They cheated to cancel out each other's cheating. And everybody believed their rivals were doing the same everywhere else in the world, from California to Kenya. Domestic championships in Russia were a farce. There were drug tests, but the very best athletes were protected and the way was cleared for them to compete at major international meets. By then they would be cleansed and ready for external inspection.

Pervakov turned out to be more than useful. He had divulged the interesting information about Melnikov's role and had brought along the relevant documentation. His bag contained a sheaf of files, all the testing plans for the National Championships, the blueprint of how those controlling Russia's athletics programme would like to be scrutinised by Rusada. He handed the forms to Vitaly.

'You might want to forward them to WADA.'

Vitaly shot him a glance. There was no reason why Pervakov couldn't forward this material to WADA himself.

Pervakov also said he had learned prior to the Vancouver Games that the Russian Ministry of Sports had a list of at least fifteen athletes — cross-country skiers, biathletes, etc. — who were untouchable. Ideally Rusada should not touch them but if requests came from WADA or elsewhere for those names to be tested, the athletes had to be informed in good time so they would have time to prepare. This list had been created by the

Russian Ministry of Sports and handed down to Director Sinev. As Pervakov was already working in the planning department, it had filtered down to him during maternity leave for his boss Natalia Vaganova. Pervakov promised to be a font of more information.

All the time, Vitaly's picture of how things worked in Russia was becoming clearer. He understood the importance of having documents that showed wrongdoing and so he became a collector. He tried not to think of WADA's reliance on the good faith of people at Rusada because that thought just sapped his energy.

Pervakov had told him another story. The detail of how it worked was unclear, but once or twice a year WADA would send each national anti-doping organisation a dirty sample that would be submitted along with the samples gathered on a regular WADA testing mission. WADA would then be informed of the result when the samples had been tested. The test was a check to make sure that a laboratory was working correctly. If everything was in order, the lab would duly test the sample and report a positive test. In Russia the agency directly responsible for testing was Rusada.

As temporary head of planning, Pervakov had been apprised of the checking system and given the task of slipping the dirty sample in with the regular samples from a testing mission. It was made clear to him that he didn't have to do anything more than that. Rusada had already told the laboratory what it needed to know. Grigory Rodchenkov had the sample number on hand and would be expecting the sample. He would, of course, report it as a positive. And so WADA could trust Moscow's anti-doping laboratory.

In one respect, all this information made Vitaly uneasy. Pervakov had casually asked him to pass documents to WADA as if everyone knew he was their go-to man. And Pervakov did not know that WADA couldn't just come to Russia and clean up the mess. It might have been useful to discuss some of these matters with Pervakov but not in the CSKA arena. Probably not anywhere actually if he was to be really prudent. He would continue to hunt but mostly as a lone wolf. He missed Oleg Samsonov, though. While not a reliable confederate, too spikily independent, he was better than nothing.

Samsonov was a bit of an enigma. An enigma who was now held in a Moscow prison. The details of why he had been arrested were hazy, as they often were in Russia, but people said a festering problem had followed him from his old job in the power industry. Vitaly had quizzed Director Sinev about it. An employee of the anti-doping agency is arrested and goes to prison and nothing is done? Everybody is vague as to what has happened? What do we know? Seriously. We must know something. He's worked here for quite some time. It can't have been something too dramatic or he would have been picked up before this.

Sinev said that Samsonov was stubborn and he hadn't behaved with the intelligence that one would have expected of a bright fellow. No matter what Samsonov thought was going to happen, this was Russia. Money opened doors easier than keys. Sinev said that if Samsonov could put together $15,000 he could walk free and get on with the rest of his life. Samsonov felt he shouldn't have to do that. He insisted that everything would be sorted out and with one stroke of a pen he would be set free, leaving the system red-faced. That was his tragic delusion. If there was anything that Samsonov could do to change his status, he was declining to do it because he didn't think he had to. It was unbecoming.

It all struck Vitaly as most mysterious. In Russia, of all places, it was more convenient and less stressful to be free than to be in jail. It was easier to fight for your name or your cause from the outside than from the inside. Yet Samsonov had decided his case should be resolved without the traditional vulgar leveraging of money or connections. For a man who knew so much about how his country worked, he seemed to have badly misunderstood his own situation.

Vitaly was concerned for him, but since the Vancouver meeting there was a new wrinkle. To the WADA delegation, Oleg Samsonov was just another Russian name. The fact that he was in prison had made no real emotional impact on them. They had no desire to meet Samsonov or to swap emails with him. What they would like to see, however, was Samsonov's notebook. Given WADA's downbeat assessment of their chances of fixing a problem like Rusada, Vitaly didn't see why. Samsonov's scribblings, if they could be located, were likely to just depress WADA even further. But if Vitaly was to provide any practical help beyond cheerleading a losing team, he had little else to offer. Since he had returned from Vancouver they'd emailed him a couple of times, asking him the same question with gentle persistence: 'Can you get the notebook?'

Samsonov had been navigating a choppy divorce before his arrest. Vitaly had come to know Samsonov's mother and girlfriend a little during the previous year. He would go and see them. He would be discreet. Find out which prison Samsonov was in and pay him a visit.

'What are you doing, Oleg?' he would ask. 'Why the hell are you still here? Are they treating you okay? And, by the way, do you still have that notebook?'

~

Back in the apartment, Yuliya simply announced that she was leaving him. Now. She was packing her things and leaving.

'You are not good for me, Vitaly. This was a mistake, Vitaly. We are divorcing.'

'Fine, Yuliya. I hope you can pack quicker than you can run.'

'Yeah? Go test yourself with your little toys and if you're happy then go and fuck yourself, Vitaly.'

He wanted to tell her to make sure to take Zina from Kursk along with the other baggage, but he sensed that Zina was actually siding with him. Zina's marriage, he learned later, was a nightmare far worse than the drama she was watching now. She could see her friend's temper and how she took out her frustration on her husband. She thought Yuliya had it good. Married to somebody sober and passive? No one gets everything. Zina's partisanship pushed Yuliya to make a better show in front of her friend, saying Zina wouldn't stick up for him if she knew.

Vitaly, meanwhile, wanted to ask his wife a question. He was at the end of his tether. Finally. He needed to know. He provided a wedding. A honeymoon. A home. Support in all things but one. He was reliable. Constant. A provider (for now anyway). Honest. Unlikely to kill any in-laws.

'Just what is your fucking problem with me, Yuliya?'

He knew the answer without hearing it, so he abandoned the conversation and walked out into the murk of a Moscow evening, not knowing if he would come back. She didn't chase him down with a teary apology.

He skulked as far as Kursky station on Zemlyanoy Val Street. He passed through the ugly modern lobby to the stately pre-revolutionary heart of the original building. Here Anna Karenina had said goodbye to Vronsky as he went off to war. The station was warm. People came and went from the busy Atrium mall across the street. Travellers stepped off long-distance trains coming from the south and north. They dashed for their metros to the suburbs or took the *elektrichka* to their dachas. Nobody went to Kursky station just to reflect. Yet the station had benches where a man could be left alone as the world scurried past, and so Vitaly took a seat.

He had been a fool. Rusada was a sham. His marriage was a

sham. What did this say about his life? Forrest Gump? He was a low-watt Walter Mitty. The daydreams he cast himself in were laughable. He wanted to be happily married to somebody who didn't want to be happily married. He wanted to be an honest employee in an organisation created by dishonesty for dishonesty. He was twenty-seven years old. It was time to be doing better. Every friend he'd had from Chelyabinsk to the United States to Moscow was pushing on with life while Vitaly was stuck on a bench in Kursky station. He was looking at being dumped from a hasty marriage and sacked from a paying job. After he'd come back from America, he'd wanted to show his parents and prove to himself that he wasn't a quitter. But now?

He sat for an hour. Two hours. Three. Four. Five.

Yuliya said she had to go. The use of performance-enhancing drugs had been built into her career plan. She couldn't show up at the track one evening and say, 'I'm not doing that any more.' 'Why not, Yuliya?' 'Because my husband said so.'

Every time she looked at him did she see judgement in his eyes? Who wouldn't want to escape that? When she won, the glory would never truly be shared. When she lost, she'd feel shattered but imagine him thinking it was for the best. She needed people around her who believed what she believed. Even he could see that. That there were no alternatives for a Russian wishing to compete.

So as he sat there, he resolved to let her go. Their marriage was like a bombed building, still standing but burnt out and empty inside. Tearing it down was the easiest solution. Move on. Do it alone. Go home again. Admit to another failure.

Once, he'd given a seminar to cross-country skiers in Syktyvkar, a city more than 600 miles north-east of Moscow. Vladimir Loginov, the vice president of the Federation, was charming. It was wonderful, he said, that Rusada was coming today. Fighting doping was good work. Yes, we have to do this, let's get this seminar rolling. Then Mr Loginov disappeared and left Vitaly to set up. In the room where Mr Loginov was they were having a few drinks – cognac, vodka and various other alcoholic beverages. Ten minutes before the start of the seminar, Mr Loginov summoned Vitaly.

'Have a small drink before your seminar so you are more relaxed.'

'Thank you, but I will be okay without it. Really.'

'No, no, you have to have it.'

'Honestly. No, thank you.'

Mr Loginov was sulky but he gave up. Vitaly inflicted his seminar on the bored and uninterested. Afterwards Mr Loginov zoned in again.

'Okay, good job, everything is good now. I am glad that you came. Let's go back to the other room. I will introduce you to some other people and then we will have a drink. Then I will take you to meet the other coaches, and we will all have dinner. Venison! But first let's go and have our drink.'

Vitaly declined politely. He was the Russian who didn't drink. All he wanted was to go back to his hotel and have a little run and just relax. He had to fly back to Moscow early tomorrow. This didn't sit well with Mr Loginov.

'It is tradition to have a drink.'

'Again. No, thank you very much.'

There were about six people standing around the table. Loginov left Vitaly in the corner and joined the group. He raised a glass in toast.

'To sport.'

They raised their glasses: 'Yes, to sport.'

'To skiing.'

They raised their glasses again: 'To skiing.'

'And to he who is not drinking because he is impotent.'

They turned to face Vitaly. They raised their glasses again.

In the Kursky station he tilted an imaginary glass and toasted his own impotency.

When he finally rose from the bench, his legs were stiff and the station was quiet. He prised the wedding ring from his finger and dropped it into a brimming rubbish bin.

It was 5 a.m. when he got back to the little apartment. In a few hours she would be gone.

Chapter 12

Yuliya was sleeping. Zina too. The women lay at angles on an air mattress as there wasn't a proper bed in the apartment. Vitaly understood that Yuliya didn't find this to be the life of her dreams. When they had argued earlier, the three of them had all been standing. It felt confrontational but there was nowhere to sit. A while ago he'd made a start at renovations. Typically, he'd had to quit. Marathons he could handle. Chores bored him. The toilet door had no lock. Everything was cold and musty. *A pair of vodka-soused drunks wouldn't live in shit like this*, he thought.

Vitaly once found himself in a church, half-listening to a Sunday sermon being given in a language not his own. The pastor was telling his flock about marriage. If you wanted to stay married for fifty years, he'd said, there were two pieces of advice: don't die and don't give up. *Amen*, thought Vitaly.

There was a night long ago when he had been woken from dreams by the sound of his parents arguing bitterly. It was strange and distressing but he couldn't drag his attention away from it. His little brother, Igor, slept on so Vitaly lay still just listening to their parents speak to each other in anger. He had never heard them like this before.

Sergey and Elena, his wildly generous parents, supported him in everything and gave him whatever he wanted. If Vitaly asked to be flown to the moon for his birthday, he knew that Sergey and Elena would find a way of launching him. He could barely remember a cross word being spoken in the house. But what did he really know of them? They had grown up in a different time and a different Russia. Their fondest wish was that things would be different and more plentiful for their sons.

Now they were hissing like vipers in a sack. They were supposed to travel to Spain together in the morning, two hard-working parents getting a break from their kids, their construction business and grey old Chelyabinsk.

His mother told his father that she knew he was cheating: 'You have another woman, Sergey.'

Vitaly waited to hear his father deny it. He didn't. His mum said that she wanted a divorce. More silence. Then more arguing. For an hour Vitaly listened to his parents go at each other. He listened until even the worry couldn't keep him awake.

The next morning his parents were up and about when he woke. They had already packed their bags and they left for their holiday in Spain with happy smiles and jaunty waves. It was as if the argument of the night before had never happened. But Vitaly couldn't unhear it. Harsh words had been traded. His mother had been hurt. His father defensive and angry. Now they were saying goodbye to Vitaly and Igor with blown kisses and see-you-soons. The workings of the big world weren't easy to understand. Vitaly was fifteen years old and wondered why he had never noticed this before. The next day Vitaly had left for America. That was all a long time ago, but his parents were still together. Not dying. Not giving up.

He lay on the floor and waited for sleep. Two hours and a buttermilk dawn passed. He listened to the familiar rhythm of Yuliya's breath.

In. He loved her.
Out. He hated her.
In. He loved her.

Was he really going to quit? Again? Probably.

Or maybe he had too many ideas about how other people should run their lives. Don't drink. Don't dope. Don't cheat. As if he was the shining path.

When he limped home in that marathon? When he stuck with Rusada till finally some wages came through? When he looked at his parents moored to each other despite everything? Had he learned anything from these things? Fight.

By 7 a.m. he had decided to go on. He would fight.

Maybe he and Yuliya weren't good for each other, but maybe they weren't so bad either. When she held his hand and jumped off the bridge into married life with him she must have felt something in that remote place she stored her affections. He wavered again as he had done all night. Then came the clarity that only a long sleepless night can bring: he would not fight at all. He would let fate decide.

At 7.20 a.m. he left the apartment again as the city was wakening to another day. He caught the subway back to Kursky station and found his platform. There was his bench. There was his rubbish bin. A cleaner hovered over the bin. Vitaly moved quickly, madness in his blood.

'Before you throw all this away, I need to look inside.'

She looked at the strung-out, saucer-eyed character in front of her. She looked at the bin filled with yesterday's mouldering crap. Was he serious? He was. He fell on the rubbish like a hungry dog. The morning chill kept the smell down, his desperation did the rest. Coffee cups, cold fries, apple cores, cigarette butts, newspapers, tissues hardened by the snot of strangers. He sifted through everything like a prospector. At last he felt the ring, the cold solid weight of it. He knew he'd found it before he saw it. This was the sign.

Back at the apartment, he told Yuliya: 'I want to keep trying.'

'You want to keep trying?' she sighed. Weary of him, though

she was just about awake. She was not impressed. She had slept on it and she was not for trying. She was for leaving.

He wanted to tell her that he had thrown away his ring. That he had rummaged through the shit and waste of Kursky station and he had found it again. It was a sign. But he knew he wouldn't survive intact past the part where he mentioned that he had thrown away the ring she'd given him.

Her stuff was packed. And Zina's face was frozen now. Then the door slammed and they were gone. So much for fate.

The championships rolled on. Two days later she failed to make the top fifteen in the 1500 metres, finishing a disappointed eighteenth of twenty-one. Vitaly didn't go to the arena but later he went to the athletes' hotel where Yuliya was staying. When he found her she had no strength left for battle. The Kursk athletes were getting ready to move out. She could go home with them and face her own people, who would see her return as failure. A career that hadn't worked out, a marriage that should never have been. Or she could stay with the loser she'd married in haste.

He sensed her vulnerability and wore her down. She really didn't want to go back to Kursk and, after making him suffer for a bit, she yielded. They hauled her stuff back to the apartment. It was early March 2010. They had been married for little more than four months. Their marriage survived only because the alternative was worse.

She told Vitaly fiercely that if he was promising to change he should start by changing in the literal sense. She really disliked the way he dressed. The successes she'd had in 2009 had brought her prize money of 120,000 roubles. They went shopping to the Evropeyskiy mall on top of the Kiyevsky subway station.

Yuliya announced the only rule of her retail therapy programme: 'I buy. You wear what I buy.'

Well, he thought, *if that's what it takes.*

She bought him jeans and shorts and things that didn't hang off him as if he was a scarecrow. She bought clothes that were tight and suggested there was an adequate body underneath. He would no longer look like a man who didn't care about how he looked. When they were done and he clutched a bag of clothes in each hand, she kissed him and whispered in his ear.

'Now you're going to fix up the apartment.'

'What about money?' he asked.

'Money is not a problem. The apartment is a problem.'

He gave himself a deadline as an incentive. His brother Igor was staying in the spare room. That could be sealed off. The rest of the apartment would be refurbished by 15 April. On that day he would travel to the US to run the Boston marathon for the second year in a row. He would see an old friend, Jared Markowitz, and for a few days he would relax.

He beat the deadline.

Chapter 13

Samsonov's girlfriend told Vitaly which of Moscow's prisons Oleg was locked up in. Vitaly planned his visit and his strategy. There were issues he wanted to sort out with Samsonov apart from custody of the notebook.

Why was Samsonov not fighting desperately to get himself out of prison? Was it fatalism or dumb optimism? Samsonov's strong suit had always been that he knew more than all those around him. It didn't seem that way any more but maybe he was holding an ace up his sleeve and waiting to play it at the right moment. And why had there been a chill between the two of them for some time? Vitaly couldn't recall any friction that might explain it. But he suspected that, before ending up in prison, Samsonov had been stockpiling information about things he saw happening in Rusada. The motivation for this was unclear but Samsonov had become secretive. Had Samsonov begun to doubt Vitaly's usefulness or was he just playing a longer game? He was aware of Rusada's flagrant collaboration with the coaches but he had gone cold on a collaboration with Vitaly. Whatever his motivation, their friendship had cooled some time before Samsonov's disappearance.

For Vitaly it was a dilemma from another time. Who to trust?

Whatever was happening with the man, Vitaly hoped Samsonov's notebook would be found to be brimming with evidence against Rusada, damning details that would be used at some future date. Or perhaps the information was already being used as a lever to blackmail those athletes and coaches whom Samsonov was apparently in constant contact with. Maybe Vitaly had seen a whistle-blower where everybody else saw a hustler. If Samsonov wanted the information to be put to good use, the right thing would be to hand it over to Vitaly. He'd lay it all out to Samsonov during the visit.

The prison building had an oppressive ugliness that advertised the unpleasantness within. At the prison reception, if that was the right word, he told the guard who he had come to see.

'Why?'

'He is my colleague and my best friend.'

'To see anybody in this jail you must be a relative. Or his lawyer.'

The guard turned his back. Conversation over. WADA would never see the notebook, and unbeknown to him Samsonov's best hope of help had been turned away at the prison door.

Throughout the rest of 2010 matters never really improved. Vitaly merely clung on at home and at work. During that summer there was major conflict between Director Sinev and the Ministry of Sports. Sinev was pushing for a little more autonomy in line with what Rusada pretended it had whenever WADA came calling. The Ministry pushed the other way, wanting total control again. Sinev versus the Ministry. There could only be one winner. One man could not stop a tank.

That summer Mr Ramil Khabriev, a well-placed official close to the Ministry for Sports, first appeared in the Rusada offices. His role was mysterious but it was rumoured he was to become Director General. A few months later Mr Nikita Kamaev turned up and he soon began running the day-to-day operations. Sinev was to be sidelined and Kamaev would become the new executive director; he and Khabriev studiously ignored all the old Rusada staff. Their presence created tension. Change was under way and people were going to get hurt.

Vitaly tried to think strategically. He made an appointment to see Konstantin Virupaev from the Ministry. He had known Virupaev from the very early Rusada days. Virupaev had been involved in the early recruitments. Vitaly knew that their meeting could be confidential and frank. Virupaev listened first in the manner of Ministry men, planning as they absorbed what you told them. He then explained the core of the problem.

Whenever Virupaev sat down with Mr Mutko, the sports minister, Mutko would tell Virupaev that in dealings with Rusada he was to make it clear that in Russia the Ministry of Sports decided everything with regard to sport. Always that was the bottom line. It didn't matter if Sinev and the others got their knickers in a twist worrying about WADA or the IAAF or the IOC. The Ministry didn't care about WADA or any other international sports bodies. 'We are in Russia,' said Mutko, 'and we live by our own rules. The Russian Ministry of Sports decides who should be sanctioned and who should be a hero and who will win the medals.' It was Virupaev's job as head of the anti-doping department at the Russian Ministry of Sports to make sure that Rusada accepted this. Rusada was a cheap shopfront for Russian sport. Rusada needed to accept this and stop complaining. Or the matter would become unseemly.

Virupaev made no attempt to sugar-coat these truths. Vitaly accepted his words as a friendly warning. Tread softly. You tread on the Ministry's turf.

Vitaly was disillusioned too with the education process that he had once placed so much faith in. Athletes slouched into seminars like school kids being punished with detention. Vitaly might have an hour to speak. His words left his mouth and floated off into that part of the ether where naivety and innocence resided. The athletes and coaches tapped away on their phones, occasionally pausing to glance at their watches. It was an ordeal for everybody. Any questions? Silence. Okay, thanks to you all for— He wouldn't even get to finish the sentence before the room had emptied.

A year after 9/11 Vitaly had packed his suitcases and left America, with regrets as his excess baggage. He'd had a special opportunity and had blown it. Yet, for some reason, each subsequent return to America revitalised him. He wasn't the best at maintaining contact but the friendships he had made could be picked up again at any time, especially with his school friend Jared Markowitz.

Jared's family had extended particular kindness in the wake of 9/11. With his apartment closed for the foreseeable future, Vitaly had been stuck. Manhattan wasn't a good place to rent and would take a while to recover. Besides that, his financial situation had worsened. The Markowitzes offered him Jared's old room while their son was at university in Pittsburgh. It meant a lot of time on buses and trains for Vitaly but the Markowitz home was a refuge. It prepared him for going home as a better person. The Russia he went home to had changed, for sure, but the air wasn't filled with the same sense of possibility that he gulped whenever he was in America. Maybe there was no such thing as the Great American Dream but there was enough of it to allow you pretend.

Jared's academic career had taken him from Carnegie Mellon University in Pittsburgh on to Massachusetts Institute of Technology, where he was doing research with MIT's highly respected biomechatronics group. Jared was involved in developing biomechanical prosthetic limbs that moved and functioned the same way human limbs do. It was unambiguously useful and satisfying work. Furthermore, Jared had become a serious runner, just as addicted as Vitaly but with a little more talent. In 2009, when they had first competed in the Boston marathon together, Jared had run 2:34:45 compared to Vitaly's 2:45:30. A year later Vitaly was consistent but nothing more, covering the course in 2:45:28, whereas Jared chopped his time down to 2:27:16. Serious running for an amateur.

To Vitaly their marathon times seemed like a metaphor. Jared's life had purpose. He knew where he was going, where happiness lay. Since Vitaly had seen Jared the previous April in Boston, he himself had been promoted and had been to the Vancouver Olympics, but he'd grown unhappy and disillusioned with his job. And there had been a sea change in Vitaly's personal life. He'd met a woman and married her within a couple of months. How could he explain this to a close friend? How could he say that already most of the time she hated him? That they threatened each other with divorce almost as often as they saw each other? One more thing. This woman I married? She's doping.

Vitaly loved his time in Boston. Jared listened without judgement and offered no pointers towards miracle solutions. Vitaly would have to make his own path through the forest.

He flew back from Boston heavy-hearted about the gloom of his domestic life and the futility of his professional life. And still he wasn't ready to give up. He had yet to answer the question that Stacy Spletzer had posed to him during the Vancouver Games: what had happened to him? He wasn't sure. Life? Love? Those things happen to most people.

As the year wore on, he found ways to spend more time with Yuliya. He separated the doping question from his wife, tucking it away for another time. He didn't want their marriage to die and, if it did, he didn't want doping to be the bridge it died on. There had been no deception. On their first date she'd told him: everybody dopes. He had somersaulted into marriage smitten with her. Something he feared he still was. He had no right to preach to her from the moral high ground. So he began to think about his words before uttering them. And he realised if he wanted a long marriage he had to play the long game.

In Rusada the more he learned the greater his fear became that things could never change. Occasionally he had to smile, so flagrant was the Russian disregard for the rules. One day David Howman, WADA Director General, and some other anti-doping people, from Norway, arrived on a visit to the Rusada offices. Some weeks before their arrival, WADA had instructed Rusada to perform an out-of-competition target test of a female boxer. While Howman and his colleagues were being schmoozed in one room by the Rusada top brass, the female boxer was in a room down the same corridor having her 'random test'. Rusada's offices had become a drop-in centre where athletes might have 'a no-notice test' at an agreed time. It amused everybody that the boxer's test coincided with the WADA visit. Russians were incorrigible.

Vitaly wrote about it later to Stuart Kemp. Told him how it was funny but not funny. He hoped that WADA would wake up and smell the roses, or the coffee, or the urine. Mainly just wake up.

He waited.

Finally, an email arrived in late June from Kemp, setting up a line of contact. Vitaly replied immediately.

From: R D
Date: Sat, 26 June 2010 at 1:00 AM
Subject: from V
To: S K

Hello, how are you? Please create a new email account (something that can't be connected to you or to your work at all, preferably not at work) and reply to me to this address and I will write to you a longer email.

Thank you. Have a great day. V. (I'm just trying to be safe, but I'll explain more in the next letter.) I'm guessing it's better to delete asap all the messages you receive from me as well.

Emails! Not the high-tech espionage device that Vitaly had hoped for, but at least somebody would be awake at the other end.

Chapter 14

Yuliya was a different beast. Vitaly watched her change. He never fully willed her to succeed but he dreaded that failure might break her heart. The National Indoor Championships had been a blow to her pride. Yet she was a girl from Kursk who had known worse things. She came back tough and hard. She got better little by little. She wore down her doubters like water dripping onto rock. People noticed her. The right people.

At the National Team Championship at Sochi that summer Yuliya surprised herself by winning the 800 metres in 2:01.99. That put her in line to represent Russia at the European Team Championships in Bergen. At the time she wasn't part of the inner circle, and those who made the decision sent Svetlana Klyuka instead. Klyuka's coach, Svetlana Styrkina, had been a champion in the 1970s and she wielded some influence.[1] Also, the decision-makers didn't know Yuliya and couldn't trust that her performance in Sochi would be replicated in Bergen. Even if it was, it probably wouldn't be good enough to win.

Neither did the National Championships bring any joy, as Yuliya finished third but missed out on a place in the team for the European Championships in Barcelona. Instead, Mariya Savinova, who didn't compete in the Nationals, was selected along with Tatyana Andrianova and Klyuka.

Not boarding the flight to Spain was a blow, but the win in

Sochi still stood as a breakthrough. Yuliya was now comfortable competing against the Moscow-based athletes who, for some mysterious reason, always seemed to have an edge on her. Better still, the national endurance coach, Alexei Melnikov, had finally begun to take her seriously. A short while before the Nationals, Melnikov had called Yuliya's coach and old lover, Vladimir Mokhnev, and asked him to enter Yuliya in the Brothers Znamensky Memorial meet, a European classic held annually in Zhukovsky, just south-east of Moscow.

With his small-town swagger, Mokhnev had called Moscow to say that Yuliya was preparing for the Nationals two weeks later and she would run the Znamensky only if Melnikov guaranteed that she wouldn't be tested. Mokhnev had overreached. Yuliya was never going to be tested at the Znamensky but the impertinence of the request wasn't well received and the conversation ended badly. Yuliya didn't compete in the Brothers Znamensky Memorial.

Then, a few weeks later, in early August, Mokhnev rang Yuliya from Kursk, saying he'd got a call from another coach.

'I have heard that there is a problem,' the other coach had said.

'Is there a problem?' said Mokhnev.

'I think, yes, that there is a problem. But for about $1,000 there will be no problem,' the other coach had replied.

Yuliya didn't understand what Mokhnev was telling her. There was an undertow of panic in his voice that made her uncomfortable.

'This guy called me,' said Mokhnev, 'but don't worry, I have a friend who knows the director of the lab.'

'And what is the problem?' asked Yuliya again. 'You haven't told me the problem.'

'EPO,' said Mokhnev.

'Shit,' said Yuliya.

A sample from Yuliya Rusanova was sitting in a lab in

Moscow and it had shown positive for EPO. Yuliya felt faint. Mokhnev continued calmly.

'You tested positive for erythropoietin during the Russian National Championships in Saransk. Look, this is not a big deal.'

But it might be. She had finished third in the 800 metres in Saransk, behind Tatyana Andrianova and Klyuka. Klyuka got silver with 2:01.77. Yuliya was clocked at 2:01.78.

She'd run a heat and a final on 12 and 13 July. She also ran the 1500 metres on the 14th and 15th – she finished fifth in the final. She couldn't even recall which day they had come for her. Now it turned out that the sample had been lying somewhere like a ticking bomb. They were teaching her a lesson because of Mokhnev's demand that she not be tested at the Znamensky Memorial. All protections had been removed. That was it, surely. She was being punished because her coach had tried to play the big guy.

'Of course it's a big fucking deal.'

Mokhnev was sort of pleased with himself, though. He was on the field with the big players now. He had called a friend who was also a friend of the lab director.

'That's right, a friend of Dr Grigory Rodchenkov. Do you know what that means?'

'No.'

'Your positive test can just disappear.'

'You know who I am married to, yes? Right. Tell me more.'

He explained. Yuliya would pay the friend of the lab director 30,000 roubles. A little less than $1,000. The friend's name was Evgeniy Evsukov. He was a very well-connected man with lots of other friends. When he got the 30,000 roubles the bad sample would disappear.

'Don't worry,' said Mokhnev. 'And, by the way, it was Russian EPO you came up positive for. The Moscow lab can detect it a lot better than any other lab in the world. So again,

DAVID WALSH

don't worry, nobody else would have detected it. They detected it and you pay money and everything will be okay. Russian EPO is still the way to go.'

She didn't like any of it. She felt cold panic. And anger. It was so unfair. Mokhnev's blithe stupidity. Everybody is doping but – because you are from Kursk and your coach is from Kursk and you are not in the golden Moscow circle – you're not protected. You can't know enough or buy enough so you get caught.

To Vitaly it all smelled strange. A shakedown? He hadn't heard anything at work in Rusada. No whispers. 'Hey, you know how Stepanov married that girl about five seconds after he met her? Well, guess what, she's tested positive.' Nothing like that. Sinev hadn't called him in to have a word in his ear. And if there was a positive in the pipeline, shouldn't there be a positive in the paperwork too? Notifications. Official procedure. Again, nothing.

Fewer and fewer things in this world surprised Vitaly, though. The more time he spent at Rusada, the more he realised how much he didn't know. As with so much of this stuff, he was out of the loop. Yuliya had told him to get his head out of the clouds. Well, this was happening. This was Russia. The test happened on home territory. Domestic testers. That was a start. Domestic troubles came with a price list. The solution was straightforward: 30,000 roubles.

As per the instructions, they got the money together in small increments instead of going to the bank and withdrawing the sum in one traceable transaction. It seemed comically cloak and dagger, but they had to play along. The instructions had been clear about that. There was to be no evidence. No holes in bank accounts, no transaction records or receipts from currency-exchange kiosks.

The handover took place at Dinamo metro station, close to the entrance. Vitaly drove them there. Yuliya got out. He

108

peered after her anxiously. When she identified the man, she handed him an envelope.

A few weeks later, good news came. Mokhnev, his credibility diminished by the EPO business, agreed with Melnikov that Dr Sergei Portugalov would help to prepare Yuliya for the 2011 winter season.[2] The bribe might be seen as a little initiation rite. A lesson about power. Never again was the EPO positive from Saransk mentioned. When you worked with Dr Portugalov, positives became a thing of the past, mishaps inflicted on ordinary people who lived outside the circle. The experience caused Yuliya to wonder if Mokhnev was the right coach for this league.

By the early winter of 2011 Vitaly sensed his time at Rusada was coming to an end. He was spiritless about the prospect. What would be, would be. Rusada would do whatever they were told by the Ministry. He was isolated at work, though still engaged with the problem of doping and the search for further evidence. He could resign, and indeed there was encouragement in that direction. But why yield to them? There was a little putsch coming and they'd find a pretext for losing whoever they wanted to lose. He doubted they'd fire him before that because he was diligent and – theoretically, at least – he would have legal redress. He was prepared to fight his corner, although there wouldn't be much point if the state was in the other corner.

On a domestic level, Yuliya was still his wife. That was a plus. In honest moments he'd admit he didn't really know how she felt about him as she focused on a career that had at last begun to blossom.

He went with her the first time she visited Portugalov in his fourth-floor office. Just one floor below them was Dr Rodchenkov and the Moscow anti-doping lab. There was a wait as Portugalov dealt with the usual queue of client athletes. When Yuliya's turn came, Portugalov shook hands with her husband in a way that made Vitaly think the good doctor had no idea who he was or what he did for a living. He was almost friendly.

Vitaly couldn't say for certain how much longer he would have a job. The Ministry men were in the offices now and those they didn't favour felt the chill of disapproval. Frozen out of everything. No hope of reprieve.

Tired of procrastination, Vitaly one day sat down and finished an email to Stuart Kemp that he'd drafted and redrafted many times since his return from Boston in April. Yuliya hadn't paused for too long about the choices she'd made. Her career came first and her marriage came second. She knew the selfishness that all athletes have. Embraced it. This had been central to the unwritten and unspoken contract between them from the start. Vitaly knew that too. He couldn't make a case for negotiating new terms more conducive to his peace of mind. He wouldn't get in the way while she outran the past. If everything that he believed to be true about sport really was true, Yuliya would have more happiness and real fulfilment if she didn't cheat. Or maybe this was just what he needed to believe.

Their arguments were circular and irresolvable. Did she think he wanted to remain married more than he wanted a wife who competed clean? Did she imagine that was his Achilles heel? The fear of losing her? If she did think that, she was wrong. He hated the sin so much there were times when he thought it would be better to just give up on the sinner.

Vitaly wrote to Kemp of his frustration and his determination.

I really wish I could prove to my wife and to people that I used to work with that doping fighting is actually a good thing to do and that it does get you somewhere. But the thing is that the only way I can show it to them besides truly believing that it is a right thing to do is if I become part of

WADA team. And I know there are a lot of people that want to work at WADA as well but, well, I still wish that. And I've been thinking about that a lot since the meeting and how far I'm willing to go. If I have to divorce my wife and be on different sides of the barricade, then I'm willing to do that. And I completely understand that she did help me to understand a lot of the things and she is just an athlete that really can't change much. And I know it's been said at the meeting that we can't change Russia but I do believe that it can be done if there is a team of people that is willing to fight for that.

What Vitaly knew was that no significant problem got solved within the plane of its original conception. He would persist and endure, and things would change, and the problem would be solved in a way not yet imagined.

For now, he existed outside of his wife. She lived in a half-lit world of secrets and lies where it was accepted that the usual conspiracy of foreigners plotted ceaselessly to do Russia down. In response Russia played the enemy at its own game and tried to play it better. Those who wondered if it was necessary to take so many drugs were asked if they imagined things were any different in rich, Western countries. As well as that, winners were appreciated and well rewarded in Russia, especially Olympic gold medallists. There was a top-of-the-range car, a classy apartment in Moscow, a good pension, sometimes a substantial one-off bonus.

Anyone who wasn't doping would have to be an idiot, and Vitaly didn't think there were many of them. He decided to lay it all out for his WADA contact as best he could. He sat down at his laptop to try once more to explain his Russia to Stuart Kemp.

Chapter 15

Sometimes Vitaly looked at himself and thought, yes, you are still an idiot. His wife's career was a positive test or a bad injury away from ending. He was about to lose his job. Yet the idea of having changed nothing gnawed at him the most. He hoped that writing to Kemp would help him untangle the web of his life, his job and his hopes. Kemp could make of it what he liked.

When he began to write, the difficulty was what to do with a problem like Yuliya. Could Vitaly claim spousal privilege and refuse to testify against his wife? Vitaly knew that if he left his wife out of the story he was telling, he wouldn't be giving the full story. Yuliya was the athlete he knew best and the woman whose involvement with doping he'd witnessed at first hand. She just happened to be his wife. That didn't make it impossible, but it was difficult. There could be consequences for Yuliya if WADA acted on the evidence he provided. He mulled over the choices and decided he couldn't exclude his wife.

He divided what he had to say into three sections: his own story, the Rusada story, and Yuliya's story. Explaining it all was the toughest part so he began with what he knew best: Yuliya. She was an elite 800 metres athlete but not part of the IAAF's registered pool of athletes, which meant she could only be tested at national championships and other high-profile track meets and while at training camps with the national team. The system made it relatively easy for her to cheat.

112

Vitaly wrote that with doping she could run 1:59 for the 800 metres, whereas without doping she ran 2:05. Doping products were bought by her coach, Vladimir Mokhnev, from a man who was a friend or business associate of Grigory Rodchenkov, the head of Moscow's anti-doping laboratory. According to Mokhnev, advice on dosages came from Rodchenkov.

Through Yuliya, Vitaly had learned how athletes can escape sanction after a positive test. Get the sample number to Rodchenkov before it is analysed, hand over 10,000 roubles (approximately $300) and the problem disappears. If the request comes after the analysis has been done, the cost is 30,000 roubles or $1,000. He related the story of how, having been secretly advised that EPO had been found in a sample of hers, Yuliya paid 30,000 roubles to make it go away, how she gave the money to one Evgeniy Evsukov, a man she'd never seen before but whom she believed was connected to Rodchenkov.

Vitaly didn't waste much time on Rusada. They had young girls out collecting drug samples whose only concern was to achieve the required number of tests. Russia's income came from conducting tests, hence the preoccupation with volume. There was no unannounced testing and no targeting of athletes whose performances invited suspicion. Only in name was Rusada anti-doping.

Finally, Vitaly talked about his own situation, which was, as so often in his life, unclear. New bosses had swept into Rusada. Change was in the air and he was one of those likely to lose his job. They'd already told him there would be no more overseas assignments. It was clear to Vitaly that they didn't trust him. That feeling was mutual, and if they fired him he wouldn't worry since the job he wanted to do at Rusada had never really existed. There were times when he felt he was being watched. Other times when it was clear someone had gone through stuff on his desk and checked his computer. What they were looking for was safely stored on the hard drive of a computer that he never took to the office.

He wrote too of the two-hour conversation he'd had with Konstantin Virupaev from the Ministry of Sport, how Virupaev had spoken with the quiet certainty of someone who knew how things worked. WADA, he'd said, wasn't really fighting doping, just playing politics. European countries were afraid of Russia. They were all just trying to stop Russia winning medals. The list of banned products was mostly politics, he'd said. Russia would always use banned products. What were the bad health consequences? He couldn't see them. The important thing was that Russian athletes were clean when they competed abroad and that there were no informers. Vitaly could do little except agree with the man from the Ministry.

And as for the notebook WADA had so eagerly sought? Well, poor Samsonov had died in prison. There was scant information regarding his demise but his plans and his hoard of information had gone with him. Vitaly put this news to Kemp in matter-of-fact terms, knowing that to WADA Samsonov was just a name and his demise meant nothing more or less than the loss of his notebook.

The Ministry had its plans, he wrote. Life would go on. No one thought anything was about to change. And that was all he could think to write. For Vitaly this was nothing more than him being true to himself. He didn't know if anybody would care or even notice, but when he pushed the send button he felt better.

Two days later Kemp's response landed in his inbox. 'Thanks for your note and for your observations. I confirm receipt of your message. Please continue to be assured that we are taking your comments very seriously and examining ways to address them in an appropriate way. Thanks for your continued support and confidence. Please stay in touch.'

No mention of Samsonov, but at least the conversation had begun.

PART TWO

'Basically the question of a drug test's results has no meaning whatsoever . . . If a test is negative it only means that the pharmacological preparation was done correctly. If it is positive then the coach is an idiot.'

Sergei Portugalov,
Head of Medical Department,
Russian Athletics Federation

Chapter 16

Three months Yuliya had spent in that wretched hospital in Kursk. She was still frail when they'd told her she could go home at last.

'You'll feel that way for another six months,' they'd said. 'Maybe longer. So avoid becoming fatigued.'

'But I'm a runner,' she'd said.

Three months was enough for illness to have stolen from her. Six more months would be cruel and unusual punishment. So she decided to train. She had bottles of pills that would keep her fighting the TB. Mokhnev said she was going to need more than that. His stock was high. In the three months she had been in hospital, Yuliya's sisters had visited her twice. At weekends she was allowed to go home, so it wasn't like they didn't get to see her. Yes, it was a long journey to the hospital, but twice? When she had been so bored.

Mokhnev had been different. He had come every other day, bearing fresh fruit. He was sweet and encouraging. He asked questions of the doctors, especially the young doctor who saw a young athlete with tuberculosis as an offence against how the world should be. They consulted regularly as to how best to beat this thing. Somebody, at last, cared about Yuliya and she was comforted by that feeling. Mokhnev had a wife and a child, but to Yuliya it mainly seemed that he had a good heart. She had bought Mokhnev's entire performance.

When their father was in prison, Katia once asked Yuliya if she might like to visit him. The answer was short and no debate followed. From his cell her dad gifted Katia the apartment he had inherited from his parents. He gave her his car too. Yuliya wanted nothing from him.

Mokhnev saw her vulnerability and worked it. He treated her well. At training camp, he taught her how to cook and clean. He told her that she would be great and special. So when she left hospital it was Mokhnev who went and spoke to her doctor about training and the recovery process. Mokhnev suggested to the doctor that things might need a kick-start.

'Prohibited substances? Is that what you are suggesting?' asked the doctor.

'Yes.'

'Yes. Yes, it would probably help with a faster recovery.'

Mokhnev started her on testosterone propionate. She didn't object.

This was what she had wanted. She had pestered him. She had asked when she felt she was reaching her limits in races beyond Kursk. She had asked about these pills she had been hearing about for some time. Could he get them or could he not? If so, could he get them for her, because she wanted to be as good as she could be? She needed to be winning.

Yes, he had said. And no. He could get the stuff. He could give it to her. Not yet, though. Her base training wasn't at the right level yet. For two years she had been running clean. This past year she had started taking vitamins and supplements. Quite a list of them, some of which required injections from Mokhnev. The list included extra iron, B12, inosine, ascorbic acid, carnitine, actovegin, mildronat, potassium orotate, glucose. She would have to wait. Now TB had made her case for doping. This was what everybody else did.

Her personal best for the 800 metres dropped in a short space of time from 2:13 to 2:08.47. Perhaps it was just the crazy self-belief she got when she was juiced. She was on a level with everybody else now. She was obsessive in her work, she had trained hard always, and now knowing what fuelled her system pushed her harder again. Drugs worked! She didn't know how they worked, but they worked.

Early in the summer of 2007 Mokhnev began administering Oral Turinabol pills and EPO injections. Yuliya's personal best duly moved down to 2:03.47 for the 800 metres. She was seventh in the Nationals for her age group. Coming off her illness the previous year and just starting out in the complicated world of performance enhancement. Seventh in the country.

She took Oral Turinabol every day for fifteen days from mid- to late May that year. The EPO she took by subcutaneous injection (of 1000 IU) every day from 30 May through to 10 June. She was still so far down the ladder that she had no unofficial licence to run dirty at the Nationals. She didn't even know such luxury existed. So Mokhnev planned the administration carefully. He had heard that Oral Turinabol would be detectable for forty days and that EPO would be detectable for nine days. Plenty of time.

When Yuliya had been in hospital the nurses would come every day to inject her. She absorbed the rudiments of the task. When she began doping, Mokhnev did the injections, but she told him that she preferred to inject herself. She understood how to do it and, knowing her own body, it just felt more comfortable. The lift that came with the drugs thrilled her. You worked so hard, but you got such a kick out of seeing your personal bests slashed time and again.

By the winter of 2007–08 she was ready to step things up again. She took a course of Oral Turinabol pills every day from mid- to late October and another course for fifteen days in February. In January 2008 she took a course of EPO injections, administering the drug to herself every other day. She also kept taking her range of non-prohibited substances. The results kept coming. The numbers kept falling. Her personal best moved down to 2:01.96. She won the National Championships in her age group and became a member of the Russian National team in the 20–23 age group.

This was working. It was happening. She was an athlete. She was winning and getting better. It was a rigged game and she was part of it now. She was a pro now. Whatever it cost her, she figured, she'd pay. She stood to gain more than anybody else. She'd come from a place that people couldn't imagine. Later she came to despise Mokhnev and his promises. His hold on her. His hands on her. He was the cost, but while she was improving she kept no track of the bill. Mokhnev could be settled at a later date.

Vitaly had written his first email to Stuart Kemp from Kislovodsk, the spa city where Yuliya had a month-long training camp. Kislovodsk was the birthplace of the dissident Aleksandr Solzhenitsyn, who wrote immense novels about state persecution. Vitaly's emails weren't going to win him a Nobel prize, or lead to eight years in a labour camp, but they too challenged the state. After returning to Moscow and thinking about what he had seen and learned in Kislovodsk, he wrote again to Kemp. There was much that needed updating.

Mokhnev had spoken with the national coach, Alexei Melnikov, about Yuliya's future. It seemed her performances had been noted and Melnikov had been waiting for Mokhnev to approach him. Melnikov worked with head of medicine, Sergei Portugalov, and the head of the Moscow laboratory, Rodchenkov. Yuliya's life was about to change.

They put her into an elite group of 800 metres runners being prepared for the European Indoor Championships in early March. Elite status came with privilege. Her medical preparation would now be overseen by Melnikov and Portugalov. Mokhnev would get the doping products from Portugalov and pass them on to Yuliya. Steroids, EPO, human growth hormone and testosterone were all more expensive now but, just as you don't quibble about the price at an upscale store, you didn't complain about the cost of membership in this exclusive athletics club.

Being in the national elite squad meant Yuliya could now compete dirty anywhere in Russia. If Rusada's testers showed up at a training camp or at a track meet, their testers would be given two lists: one showing the athletes they could test, the other showing those they couldn't test. Every two to three weeks, elite athletes had blood and urine analysed so that Portugalov and Melnikov knew when it was safe to allow their athletes to be tested.

And in other news, things at Rusada had got worse. Ramil Khabriev, the new executive director, didn't spend much time in the office but word filtered through that the new boss didn't think much of the staff he'd inherited. Director Sinev was blamed for the inefficiency. A few days before the end of the year, everyone was informed about a restructuring of the agency that would be in place from 1 March 2011. At that point, every job would be advertised and the different criteria for each position would be posted on the website. Vitaly realised that few of the current staff would be well enough qualified under the new requirement. His time at Rusada was almost up.

Vitaly also told Kemp that he thought Yuliya would have a better year in 2011, now that her doping was being supervised by the All-Russia Athletic Federation (ARAF). It wasn't a prospect that excited or even pleased him. Conflicted, he tried to explain his predicament.

'I'm not making any kind of excuses,' he wrote, 'but sometimes I talk with my wife and I tell her that her health is more important for me than anything else but the fair questions that she asks me:

Do you want me to quit running? Do you want me to give up on my dreams? I can't make her quit and I hope you understand that this doping system was here for the past forty years or so and it might take a lot of time for people to change their mindset and start trying to do things the honest and fair way.'

As for Portugalov, well, most coaches extracted the potential of an athlete like men pushing toothpaste from a tube. They squeezed until nothing was left. Then they got a new tube to squeeze. Portugalov was different. Portugalov replenished and restored you.

It was December 2010 and Yuliya was now part of the magic circle. First Portugalov established ground rules, the client/supplier conditions:

1. Better if you don't bring your husband around again.
2. Do what you are told.
3. Cash only.

He wanted to know her history with doping. 'You took what? Who told you to take that? How much? Why?' He frowned like a man once again reminded of how many imbeciles operated in his area of expertise.

Her previous experience had been of Mokhnev haphazardly loading her up with substances that he obtained from goodness knew where and that he understood little about. The packages didn't come with easy-to-use instructions but, even if they had, Mokhnev's arrogance would have prevented him from reading them. He worked like a man trying to assemble a car without instructions or adequate tools. Sometimes he got lucky. Sometimes he didn't. When Yuliya worried aloud about the effects the drugs were having on her body he had no answers. His interest in her body didn't lean that way. He waved her concerns away with the breeziness of the bluffer.

She told Portugalov how Mokhnev would divide a 2ml testosterone ampoule into seven equal parts, then inject each one-seventh part under her skin every third day. Portugalov smiled and shook his head.

'Testosterone injections are good only when the ampoule has just been opened.'

She felt embarrassed for Mokhnev. Only a fool divided the ampoule into seven parts. The first part actually did something. The other six parts quickly became a placebo. When you needed to protect something from air and contaminants, you might use ... an ampoule. That was the clue right there.

'By the way,' Portugalov added, 'testosterone is used for intramuscular injection only. Not under the skin.'

She knew Portugalov was right, but even the incorrectly administered one-seventh of an ampoule had done its work heroically. She looked forward to what Portugalov would deliver.

On Mokhnev's improvised regime her muscles had sometimes tightened so much that she had to stop running. Tests occasionally showed that her haematocrit and haemoglobin levels were too high. Too many red cells thickened the blood, which could be dangerous. Ignorance being bliss, Mokhnev was content with everything. She had heard the stories of cyclists who had used EPO until their blood clogged their hearts. Cyclists who died in their sleep. The stories were old but they had the power to haunt her. But the more she improved, the less she worried. She'd kept on training through her anxieties, injecting Trental, a medicine for occlusive heart conditions, whenever she needed to thin her blood. Such was her flimsy protection against the recklessness of her coach.

She told Portugalov how Mokhnev had done things. He shook his head slowly as he listened.

'Yuliya,' he said, 'other athletes don't go through weeks with stiffened leg muscles. Did you think that was normal? This man

Mokhnev lacked the basic knowledge to protect you. You could have died.'

After the first season they hadn't done much tampering with her doping regime. Nothing seemed broken, so why tinker? They branched out a little with oxandrolone and Parabolan. Things Mokhnev had heard about. In the real world, people thought taking so many drugs must be a rodeo ride for the body, but she found things to be smooth and cyclical. The more she trained, the more pharmacological help she needed to keep improving.

Now, as Portugalov reminded her, she was working with a professional. He restated rule number two: just do what you are told and everything will be good. Oh, and one more rule: make sure you always keep clean frozen urine in the freezer for unforeseen situations arising from unplanned encounters with non-Rusada doping controls.

She took the new drugs mainly in winter and spring. By the time it came to the business end of the year she would be fettled like a racehorse. Being a Portugalov client was such an upgrade, it felt like turning left when you boarded a plane. You were tended to and pampered. There were decent athletes huddled back in economy, just-glad-to-be-there types, but up at the front cabin of Russian sport were those who were chosen by Portugalov. The small worries of the ordinary athlete weren't for them.

'Yuliya,' Portugalov said, 'I want you not to worry about running dirty at the National Championships. You *will* be running dirty at the National Championships. Okay?'

She wasn't sure if a big thank-you was the appropriate response. 'Okay.'

When they tested her at the Nationals all she needed to do was text Portugalov her sample number. Then she just had to get on with her day. She had entered a new world.

In the weeks that followed, she noticed that some people from Nike began to say hello. They stopped by and shook her hand. They were hearing good things, they said. She was a special runner, they said.

At the 2010 National Championships Yuliya had finished in third place, missing selection to the Europeans in Barcelona by one hundredth of a second, the breadth of a fine hair. At that time Portugalov's fine tuning was still in her future. He needed only to apply the finishing touches. One hundredth of a second? It was nothing. He could give you that just by allowing you to sit in his waiting room and breathe the air.

She called him The Professor. He was omniscient and wise. The proof of that came soon enough. Early in 2011 she ran a 600 metres race in 1:24.02 (just .58 off the seven-year-old world record) during the Russian Winter IAAF Indoor Meet in Moscow. Mariya Savinova, the World Indoor 800 metres champion, was using the race as a warm-up for the outdoor season and finished second in 1:26.23. Afterwards Portugalov told Yuliya that she would run 1:55 for the 800 metres in London at the 2012 Olympic Games. At the time her personal best was 1:58.99, so 1:55? Could he be serious? Did she have that in her? She wasn't sure, but she knew one thing: she was going to adhere to rule number two.

~

Alas, poor Samsonov. Questions had lingered after his death. It was said that he had died in prison from a heart attack. There was no alternative to the official version because exploring your own theory was nigh on impossible. Certainly Samsonov's health had been imperfect. The circumstances of his committal to prison and his reluctance to explore the possibility of getting out and returning to his job and girlfriend were unexplained. Sometimes Vitaly would think that Samsonov knew too much.

After the Beijing Games, Rusada had moved into more expansive offices over the Kiyevsky metro station. One of the rooms was like a smallish conference room, enough space for maybe ten desks, and one wall served as a giant screen onto which presentations or films could be projected. Samsonov had commandeered this space. He procured high-definition videos of all the athletics finals from Beijing. He studied them compulsively. The most unbelievable thing had happened with the Russian female team in the 4 × 100 metres relay: the Jamaicans had dropped the baton and the Americans had been sanctioned, so the Russians had won the Olympic gold.

Samsonov enjoyed the irony of it. So unexpected. But he kept showing Vitaly the Russian male performance in the 4 × 400 metres. The runners did really well but there was one runner Samsonov kept pointing to. His personal best was something like 46 seconds, and in that relay in the final he'd run something in the region of 44.5. Maybe a second and a half faster than his best. Samsonov's inquisitive face had stayed with Vitaly. He often wondered what would happen if the IOC opened those particular Beijing samples years later. Most of the athletes in Russia were said to be on stanozolol at the time. Surely new testing methods would settle the question that Samsonov seemed to ask.

Why would a clever man choose to remain in prison rather than muster the money to slip into somebody's back pocket? Director Sinev had said that financial help had been offered to Samsonov. $15,000 would do it. Had that help been offered officially or unofficially? Or at all? Sinev never elaborated. Did Samsonov think the secrets he carried in his black notebook made for better leverage? That with the information he had he was somehow bulletproof? Nobody would ever know.

Otherwise the war stories from DCOs were still the same narratives of dismissal and despondency. The culture of Russian sport wasn't changing in any way Vitaly could detect. He wished he knew a little bit more about the rumoured second laboratory that was run, it was said, by a friend of Dr Grigory Rodchenkov. People said the lab was paid for by the city of Moscow. Why? Nobody knew.

~

Yuliya continued to do well in spring 2011, showing instant improvement under Portugalov's care. After the 600 metres success she took the 800 metres title at the Russian Indoor Championships in February, finishing in 1:58.11 ahead of Yevgeniya Zinurova in 1:58.83 and Elena Arzhakova in 1:59.35. It was a new personal best, and electric form for February. The first three to cross the line qualified for the European Indoors in Paris two weeks later. This was a giant step towards the big time. She was finally representing Russia at a championship meeting. A trip to Paris! The feeling of real power in her legs. Vitaly tried to share her excitement but he couldn't quite pull it off.

The deeper she went into the world that Portugalov had opened up for her, the more she learned. The dates when you needed to have your system clean by were pushed back to later than she had ever imagined. She loved the confidence of those inside the system, their brinkmanship with the world anti-doping people, the depth of knowledge underlying it all. These guys had been doing this for ever. They had started out in a different Russia, a Russia she never knew. They had been the constant thread of the nation's sports from the Soviet time to the oligarch era. They made champions for a living. Being part of their world, she felt different about herself. It was like her self-esteem was on one end of a see-saw, her 800 metres times on the other end. And they had accepted her. They weren't in the business of training donkeys for derbies. They worked with thoroughbreds. The better you were, the more protection you got from them. The more protection you got, the more chemical assistance you could take. It was a beautiful cycle.

She would explain these things to Vitaly, telling him to be happy for her. If he was going to be her husband, he was going to have to enjoy her success. He smiled and nodded and tried to hide his discontent. The words he had written to Kemp about his willingness to seek a divorce swam in his mind. It seemed his own world of anti-doping activity hardly trespassed into Yuliya's consciousness. All his thoughtful parables about morality, ethics and health were stuff she didn't think had much relevance to elite-level sport. Now in Portugalov's circle, she knew that to be the case.

Vitaly had other outlets for his frustration.

Chapter 17

When Vitaly came home with some news of his own, there was no joy to be shared. Bad tidings but not unexpected. The sword had finally fallen. He was out of work. Discarded as part of the regime change. He came back to his desk one day and found an envelope waiting for him. Without having to open it, he guessed its content.

Nobody had ever come and told Vitaly that he would be fired, but he had guessed long ago that his name would be high on the list drawn up by Mr Khabriev and Mr Kamaev. The clue was in the failure of either of them to say a single word to him for six months. It hadn't augured well. Before that there had been little motivational chats. Hints dropped. Everybody hoped Vitaly would perk up. Go with the flow. Just be a little more flexible. Why make people in the federations uncomfortable? The Ministry doesn't like people in the federations being uncomfortable. Who would? They weren't all bad people, Vitaly. Work with us. Work with them. Just try not to be so uptight about it all. This is Russia. Even in the darkest days we had ways around rules.

For a while everybody had felt threatened. The winnowing took place in the traditional way. Those who would save themselves surrendered their dignity first. Vitaly watched Derevoedov and Zagorskiy sweet-talk Kamaev into believing they knew what was happening and that he needed their support. It worked for them. When Kamaev sat down with the task of deciding who would stay in Rusada and who would go, the two people sitting nearest to him were Zagorskiy and Derevoedov. They contributed to the debate.

The Rusada travel department had recently informed Vitaly – on 20 February, to be precise – of the sample collection and educational seminars he would be travelling to in March. He had signed all the papers for travel but he knew it meant nothing. The travel department weren't in the loop either. In the end nobody said anything. He just came back to the office after lunch and there was the envelope on his desk. 'We looked at your qualities and unfortunately we cannot offer you anything with your qualities.' And that was it. Sinev was gone too.

Vitaly shared the news with Stuart Kemp, who he was coming to regard as an agony aunt who didn't always respond to problems. As matter-of-factly as he could, he told the story of his firing and described how Rusada had changed. Ramil Khabriev didn't know that much about anti-doping and it seemed to Vitaly that the new regime weren't very interested in upholding the WADA code. As for his own situation, he was now an anti-doping advocate without a platform. If there was a way to continue this work he would welcome any help, but he added that he expected nothing. His wife, on the other hand, was going from strength to strength, running faster and faster under Portugalov's tutelage. The difference now was that she was part of the system. Towards the end of his email, Vitaly said he wanted Kemp to understand that if her rivals in Russia were competing clean, Yuliya would happily do the same. He signed off by asking Kemp to acknowledge receipt of his email. It sounded like a plea for help.

~

Yuliya had met with Portugalov for the first time before heading to a training camp in Portugal. When she returned they met again. It was late December. He had devised the formula she needed. She was taken aback at first. It sounded like the doping regime of a racehorse. Three injections (half an ampoule each) of testosterone. She had her doubts but she wasn't paying money to second-guess the master. She injected herself as required on 29 and 31 December and again on 3 January.

He gave her oxandrolone, an old-school anabolic steroid particularly suitable for women, its impact being more anabolic than androgenic. She was to dose herself with this when the three big testosterone injections were done, so she took it from 3 January for three weeks. From 10 January he started her on a course of EPO injections of 2,000 units/ml each day. She had previously just dipped her toes into the EPO sea with some 1,000 units/ml shots. With the EPO, he recommended she inject Venofer, a substance that counters iron-deficiency anaemia.

Her body responded unquestioningly. Felt stronger. Allowed her to run faster.

Next, Portugalov told her to take one ampoule of testosterone and not to do any hard workouts for three days as she could tear her muscles. By now his word was her command. This was what athletes paid money for. Everywhere in the real world – and the real world didn't end at Russia's borders – this was how athletes prepared. Real athletes. More stuff and better stuff. You were training hard but you also were training smarter. That translated into milliseconds, which were cashed in for medals. You could spend the best years of your life being a fool and an also-ran or you could be smart and make the most of the opportunity nature had given you. She believed that only now was she starting her career. Everything else had just been part of a tortuous journey to this point.

She did a couple more EPO injections in the days after the

600 metres run. She took the second injection on 10 February along with a last half-ampoule of testosterone.

On 16 and 17 February she competed at the National Indoor Championships, winning her heat with a time of 1:59.98 and then the final in 1:58.14. After the final she was tested by Rusada, but with her new status the post-race test was a protocol, not a problem. When she left the doping control station she pulled the pink copy of the doping control slip out of her pocket and texted her sample number to Portugalov.

Her sample tested negative. As did all the samples of athletes preparing seriously for the Europeans in Paris a few weeks later. Though Yuliya knew she was protected, she still felt some anxiety until the result came back. She supposed that in time one just came to take this service for granted.

A week before Paris, Rusada tested everybody all over again. Nothing to be alarmed about. These are the 'away' tests. A precaution. The Ministry demands away tests before any meetings abroad in order to minimise the chance of an embarrassing cock-up. Rusada would ensure all the doping athletes would actually be clean when they got to Paris. It was a silly procedure that everybody went through before competing internationally, she was told. If you failed the away test, you would get tested again a day or two later. If you failed the second away test, you stayed home. Simple. Russia has its reputation to think of.

She wasn't ready to take any chances. Home or away. A day or so after she qualified she went to Portugalov again and asked for specifics about what she should do between then and Paris. This was fresh territory. How to clean one's system without losing too much required a degree of precision she had never thought possible. What was safe? Suppose her metabolism had some kink? She needed to get this right. Portugalov laid out the plan with no fuss. The away tests were just a gateway on the path to Paris.

'We'll reduce certain doses and we'll continue with other drugs,' he said, 'but in the end you should know, Yuliya, that I am making bets with my friend Grigory Rodchenkov and other people. I have bet money that you will win in Paris.'

She told Vitaly about Portugalov's optimism. He nodded. *Now they're wagering on my wife as if she is a racehorse*, he thought.

Yuliya didn't win in Paris; she was third, in a time of 2:00.80 behind Yevgeniya Zinurova's 2:00.19 and the British Jenny Meadows' 2:00.50. Yuliya's time from two weeks previously would have won her gold. Here, though, Meadows had dominated for 700 metres. In the last half-lap Zinurova had glided confidently through the field and reeled in Meadows in the final metres. Yuliya closed fast for her bronze medal but she was never really part of the central drama. The quote she gave to the media afterwards reflected something of her confusion.

'It was a difficult race. I expected it to be easier even if I knew that Jennifer will run very fast from the start. I was nervous and there was too much responsibility on my shoulders. I tried to catch Jennifer before the finish but did not have enough power. Now I am looking forward to a good sleep and a relax.'

In France on 3 March she gave blood for her blood passport for the first time. Her results were Haemoglobin (Hb) – 16.1, Haemocrit (Ht) – 48.5, Reticulocyte count (Re) – 0.31, Off-score (Off-s) – 127.6. The haemocrit is the ratio of red-blood cells to total volume of blood in the body. Reticulocytes are immature red blood cells without a nucleus. Haemoglobin is the oxygen-carrying protein carried in red-blood cells to the muscle. Blood doping and EPO increase the amount of haemoglobin in the blood. The key readings in the biological passport are reticulocytes and haemoglobin, which are combined statistically to produce an Off-score or 'stimulation index', a ratio of haemoglobin to reticulocytes. The Off-score can suggest both withdrawal of blood (a rise in reticulocytes and a decline in haemoglobin) or a re-infusion of blood (reticulocytes decline and haemoglobin rises). In healthy non-doping athletes none of these values fluctuate much.

She tested as abnormal! An off-score of over 103 in a female athlete can trigger investigation or targeted testing, now Yuliya had appeared on the radar. She had one strike against her name. So too had Portugalov and Melnikov. The salient details of the passport programme and the danger it represented for doping athletes had yet to be fully understood by some of the most influential figures in Russian athletics.

She came home from Paris with her medal. It was a first international medal for her but Vitaly wanted no part of it. Not because it was bronze but because it was stolen. In Kursk, though, a bronze medal at the European Championships was a big deal. Journalists came to interview her and her family. But Vitaly told her he would not be there, he would not be in on it. He was still the man who wouldn't drink or dance at his own wedding.

London 2012 was now on her horizon. She could feel her growing strength. Vitaly found it hard to celebrate her achievements, she got that. But he didn't have a job now and she was the breadwinner. And as Portugalov plotted her immediate future, nothing was going to distract her.

∼

In April 2011 Vitaly returned to Massachusetts for his third consecutive Boston marathon. The result of his friendly rivalry with Jared went unchanged. Jared ran 2:26:37 while Vitaly came home in 2:43:53. Vitaly wondered what his friend would run if Portugalov was in his corner.

Vitaly would remain in Boston for two days of meetings with WADA personnel. He discussed the matter privately with Jared. The talk reminded them both of the divergent paths they had taken since first meeting in Pennsylvania almost fifteen years earlier. Jared didn't give much advice other than for Vitaly to just be careful.

Vitaly was at a fork in the woods. He'd written a line to Stuart Kemp: 'Life definitely would have been different if I didn't drive you from the airport in Moscow in 2008.'

By now WADA offered the only possible exit from the mess Vitaly was in. They would have a small group staying at the InterContinental on Atlantic Avenue, the kind of big, shiny, bland hotel that elite sports officials favoured. Vitaly let them know he would be at Jared's place in Cambridge. If they called, Jared would answer.

Vitaly met the WADA delegation on the evening of the marathon. The surroundings were fine, the hosts painstakingly welcoming. 'Do you need to eat, Vitaly? More water? More coffee?' In Jack Robertson, WADA's chief investigations officer, Vitaly sensed a vivid, cinematic past. Olivier Niggli was the agency's intense and quietly spoken legal and finance director. And there was Julien Sieveking, a legal expert who was fair-haired and assured and, like Niggli, a Swiss lawyer. He seemed to work for Niggli and deferred to him. Stuart Kemp was the fourth member of the delegation.

After the brief introductions, Jack Robertson was the one Vitaly was most intrigued by. Robertson seemed like the real deal, with two decades working for the US Drug Enforcement Administration (DEA) mostly in the borderlands south of San Diego. He had a resumé full of blockbusters: Operation Cardinal Sin (the one with the Arellano-Félix Organization, or Tijuana Cartel), Operation TKO (Mexico again, the one with the ketamine and steroids), Operation Gear Grinder (the one with Mexico and more steroids), Operation Raw Deal (the USA this time, the one with even more steroids), Operation Counter-Curse (the one with the USA, Canada and the synthetic drugs),

Operation Motley Crew (the one with the return of the Tijuana Cartel). One year his colleagues voted him 'Agent of the Year'. Not bad when there were five thousand agents to choose from.

That evening and all the next day, over endless food and coffee, they combed through the detail of Vitaly's correspondence with Kemp. All the time they wanted more detail, more names, more background. The past. The future. Big players. Small players.

The second lab in Moscow was the subject of many whispers within Rusada. Fine. But does it exist? Why do you think so? Okay. Your wife Yuliya and Portugalov? How's that? How does the system operate for individual athletes? Athletes pay coaches as a matter of course for drugs. Okay. How? Cash? Card? Gift tokens? Details, details, details. Who does the coach pay? Is this just hearsay?

They took lots of notes. They made noises and words. 'Hmm.' 'Interesting.' 'Really? Wow.' They exchanged glances. They exhaled wonder. They never said, 'Okay, Vitaly, here's the plan.' Or: 'Okay, Vitaly. We are going to take it from here.' One thing became clear: this river of information was very interesting to WADA but useless too. It irrigated nothing. They were appreciative of Vitaly's courage in coming forward, but it seemed they were still tied by cuffs of their own design.

Vitaly didn't doubt their sincerity but it became clear they weren't able to help. It was depressing and disheartening. WADA had been created with its own assumption undermining it. There would be no more state-sponsored cheating. True? Doping had moved into the era of privatisation. Governments would never travel that road, not after the fall of the German Democratic Republic's sport empire. If there was a problem anywhere in the world, WADA would alert the anti-doping authorities in the local precinct. Simple? Nobody had imagined that the anti-doping police might be as corrupt as the place they policed. Nobody had made contingencies for a rogue state. WADA's delegation had come from Montreal to hear chapter and verse on Russia cheating, but the most important realisation was that they couldn't do anything about it.

'Unfortunately we have to tell you that the only people who can investigate Russian institutional doping are Russian institutions.'

Vitaly knew what that would lead to.

'Thank you. Goodbye,' they said, shaking his hand and making eye contact. 'Listen, you be careful.'

By the time he touched down on Russian soil, Vitaly viewed the glass as half-full again. Jack Robertson? Vitaly sensed he'd been to places, seen things, done things. The kind of man who, when you told him there was nothing more he could do, he wouldn't always agree.

Chapter 18

Back in the den of the bear, Vitaly was freshly jobless but still married. He had heard unemployment approaching but he'd been unable to avoid it. He wouldn't make the same mistake with divorce. He had time now and he gave it to Yuliya. They travelled together to training camps in Portugal and to Lake Issyk-Kul, 1,600 metres above sea level in Kyrgyzstan, where your lungs took a while to get used to reduced rations.

The Russian National Championships in Cheboksary in late July were the last chance for Yuliya to make the national team for the World Championships in South Korea a few weeks later. She slaved during training and did exactly as she was told by Portugalov when off the track. The women's 800 metres competition would be pressure-cooker intense. Russia had a deep pool of talent that the rest of the world envied. What happened in Cheboksary would be studied by coaches, athletes and experts everywhere. In the 800 metres Russia's women were the superpower. Only the top two women from the superpower would be on the plane to South Korea. As was the custom, the council of coaches had the right to add a third name if there was an athlete they deemed worthy. They could choose somebody who, for good reason, hadn't even taken part in the National Championships, but the practice was for the third-place finisher to get the berth.

Yuliya travelled to Cheboksary with the confidence of a

woman who knew her time had come. This would be the proving ground for Portugalov's work. She wouldn't disappoint him.

In the preliminaries the reigning World Indoor and European Outdoor 800 metres champion, Mariya Savinova, stood out.[1] She posted 1:58.03 in her heat. A searing run for this time of the year. Only three other runners ran below the two-minute mark under the blazing yellow sun: Elena Kofanova (1:59.14), Svetlana Klyuka (1:58.70) and Yevgeniya Zinurova (1:59.94) were flying.[2] The qualifiers would surely come from that group.

On the start line for the final, Yuliya noted that seven of the other finalists had gone under two minutes during the season. Good for them. She herself had shown nothing in getting here. Nobody who searched online that evening for the result of the Russian 800 metres final was surprised to see that Savinova had taken gold. She improved once again in the final, posting her outdoor personal best of 1:56.95. Mariya Savinova wasn't the story, though. She had needed to bust a gut to cross the line ahead of a runner from Kursk who had run her own personal best of 1:56.99 right when it mattered. Those who took an interest in the sport were getting to know the young woman who still raced under her maiden name, Yuliya Rusanova.

Behind Yuliya, Yekaterina Kostetskaya finished third in 1:57.17, ahead of Klyuka in 1:58.03 and Kofanova in 1:58.25.[3] At the end of the race, the four fastest 800 metres runners in the world for the season were Russian. The first three were duly selected for Daegu.

Yuliya's time confirmed that she had made the right choice when she had paid her money to Portugalov. London 2012 was a year away. Perhaps even a 1:55 was now possible.

~

After Boston, little changed in Vitaly's sterile relationship with WADA and Stuart Kemp. He continued to send emails and drummed his fingers as he waited for some plan of action to emerge from the world's anti-doping police. Kemp's position was, in retrospect, a little difficult. At the other end of an email correspondence with the likeable lunatic who had driven him through Moscow a couple of years previously, he was not in a position to do anything other than offer his gratitude, gentle advice and encouragement. Like everyone else at WADA, he was hemmed in by the agency's own rules and was mindful too of the ethical dilemma. He was in no position to push Vitaly into places where he or Yuliya might be put in danger. For that matter, neither could he afford to play fast and loose with his own job by swerving WADA rules. The limits of what could be done had been clear to him for some time, but it made no sense to cut Vitaly off. He appreciated the quality of the information coming through and the sincerity of the man who pushed the send button every time. The paralysis at WADA would have to be dealt with imaginatively.

Sometimes Vitaly's correspondence with Kemp was just a clearing house for bits and pieces of gossip. At other times it was a valve that permitted Vitaly to get things off his chest. He was out of the loop since losing his job, though he had not been integral to the loop before that. A feature of his trips to Beijing and Vancouver had been hearing tales of Rusada's misdemeanours from other people.

One evening in Beijing back in 2008, he had found himself with Chris Butler, an Australian who worked in France for the IAAF. Butler was good company. They spoke about Russia. Vitaly had told a story about travelling to the race-walking centre at Saransk in Mordovia to do unannounced testing on the walkers not long before the Games. He had been met at the station by two minions and a BMW dispatched by Viktor Chegin, Russia's race-walking guru. Just a reminder that the random visit of a doping control officer was no surprise to a made guy like Chegin. Later Vitaly, having declined a cosy offer to share some caviar and a sauna, was left to make his own way back to the station.

While he was in Saransk Vitaly had had the sense of being watched. He was used to the shunning by then and forgot about it but, a week before Beijing, Chegin had made an announcement that caught Vitaly's attention.[4] Chegin had trained a local hero, Valeriy Borchin, since 2004, sticking with him through a year-long ban after a positive for ephedrine. Now Borchin and fellow racer Vladimir Kanaykin seemed to have failed random tests back in April. EPO was mentioned. Kanaykin dropped out of the Beijing Games, apparently of his own accord, but Borchin claimed to know nothing of any positives and brazened it out. There was no suggestion that that his own federation might ask Borchin to withdraw.[5]

The Russian team travelled to Beijing with luminous questions marks on their backs. Seven serious Russian medal prospects had received doping bans on the eve of the Games. It was a large elephant to have in any room. Valentin Balakhnichev, president of the All-Russia Athletic Federation (ARAF), said that he was mystified by it all. Hurt and mystified. Russia had no choice for now but to comply, but in due course Russia would be looking into it further.

Vitaly knew the audience Balakhnichev was playing his song to. So many Russians believed that beyond their borders a malevolent 'they' was waiting in the tall grass with nothing else in mind but doing Russia down. The driving passion of this conspiracy was the sense that it was better for Russia to lose a race than for any of the conspirators to win. Russia's suffering was the reward. Everything else was bonus. If a person knew this to be true, that person knew nothing bad was ever Russia's fault. That was how it was. With their banning of seven Russians before Beijing, those tricky foreign do-gooders had pulled the rug from under Russian feet again. Pure jealousy.

Butler had given Vitaly a different version of the world. Earlier in the year an international doping control officer had travelled to the Russian National Championships in Kazan to take the DNA samples that would become central to the case. People from Rusada had been present at the testing. Saliva samples had been taken. Everybody from Rusada to Balakhnichev had known exactly what was coming down the tracks. And why. Vitaly was stunned. If it was well known in Rusada, that meant Director Sinev knew. All the times Vitaly had collected Sinev to drive him to the office, all the times he had driven him home again while chatting about the events of the day, yet not a word.

Better understanding his limitations, Vitaly was happy to keep the information supply lines open and to just hope for the best. Surely something would change. As for Kemp, sometimes when he panned through the information he found useful little nuggets.

As spring of 2011 approached, Vitaly mentioned in passing a situation concerning a man who would later feature in many emails and conversations, Grigory Rodchenkov. He'd heard that on 24 February agents from the federal drug enforcement department had discovered that Rodchenkov's wife had been caught selling steroids. Here, Vitaly's information was incorrect. It had been Rodchenkov's sister Marina who had been implicated in selling performance-enhancing drugs. She would be sentenced to eighteen months in prison, later suspended. Vitaly explained that Rodchenkov had fallen ill after Marina's arrest and been hospitalised. Two officers from the drug control service had turned up at Rusada's office looking for Sinev, who was no longer at the agency.

A short while later, Kemp wrote to Vitaly. He cited an odd

email that had come to WADA, full of grammatical solecisms and a fascinating rumour. Intriguingly, this was a different version of the Grigory/Marina story; different details but essentially the same narrative. There was enough confidential information in the email to suggest it came from someone on the inside. The emailer added one important detail: after the opening of the investigation, Grigory had tried to kill himself and was now in a special clinic. The investigation was continuing. Official Russia was doing its damnedest to keep the story out of the public domain.

Vitaly was pleased that somebody else was shining a light into dark corners. He promised Kemp he would visit Rusada on a fishing expedition to see what his former colleagues might say about it all. Moscow was usually a good city for deep gossip and Vitaly was sure that, among the surviving Rusada staff, he would find one soul who was as disaffected as he had been. He also sent Kemp some links to Russian websites that were humming with versions of the Rodchenkov business. He expressed his surprise at the information being so 'out there'. When he visited Rusada, however, his old colleagues knew nothing fresh about the Rodchenkov story. Websites were their source of information too. The one thing Vitaly learned was that Rodchenkov wasn't signing any official documents from the lab. Wherever he was – hospital or special clinic or wherever – he wasn't in his lab.

Nothing more than that. Dead end. Like a spring snow, the Rodchenkov story vanished, even if the memory survived.[6]

~

Vitaly travelled with Yuliya to Daegu in South Korea. There was unease among the coaches when they learned he would be travelling with them. He was no longer the square peg in the Rusada round hole, but he was still a piece of unwanted baggage. Not to be trusted. Melnikov was insisting to Mokhnev that Vitaly could not go. No way. Stop it. Mokhnev agreed but there was nothing he could do. The good old days, when others would decide where loose ends like Vitaly could travel, were gone and missed. Everybody would just have to live with it. This was the world now.

The trip was a disappointment. Having run 1:56.99 to qualify, Yuliya was confident that she could compete for a medal. She didn't say it out loud because she knew her place, but in her heart bronze would be a disappointment.

She ran horribly in the heats and hoped her form would emerge in the final. It didn't. She finished last with a plodding 1:59.74. Mariya Savinova ran 1:55.87 for the gold. To have turned in such a qualifying time only to be so far off the pace in a world final was a kick in the gut. She had trained hard. She had focused. She had taken every pill and injection she was offered. Why had Savinova stayed at her own level while Yuliya had gone backwards? How was that done?

As she did the forensics on her loss, it emerged that for some athletes there was a category of service beyond first class. Portugalov, it seemed, worked differently with different athletes. Savinova, for example, was in a category that might be called 'first class plus'. She enjoyed those little extras that made the difference. She was being provided with more help and this was what she paid extra money for. It was help that continued right to the eve of a big race.

Both Yuliya and Savinova had qualified for the Worlds from the same race in Cheboksary but, from that point until Daegu – and indeed in Daegu itself – Yuliya's doping regime was limited to AndroGel, a testosterone gel that safely cleared the system in a day. Savinova had been on a mixed diet of peptides, human growth hormone and other unspecified products to keep her engine revved and ready. Portugalov had made sure she was constantly monitored. Private doping tests were administered every day. Savinova was the horse in the stable who was trained to win. Yuliya had been trained to make the podium. The bottom line was Savinova was paying more money and Savinova was winning. It stood to reason, therefore, that she was making a lot more money than Yuliya. The system fed itself.

The problem seemed obvious to Yuliya. Russia had, for instance, a constellation of 800 metres runners. Portugalov couldn't offer the top eight of these runners his 'first class plus' service. There were only three medals to be won. Somebody was going to finish last, no matter how much help they had injected and ingested. Or maybe he was that cynical. Maybe you just had to ask and stump up more money. What was he doing, after all, but giving each girl the best chance to achieve? After that it was hard work and natural talent that made the difference. That's what every girl had realised way back when somebody had given her the talk about wising up. 'They' were all doped up to their tanned Californian asses, their lily-white English necks, their dark Jamaican eyes. Only an idiot would have the arrogance to think she could run for Russia on fresh air and healthy food.

Except Yuliya didn't truly believe that. Not in her heart. Not in her soul. Not the week after the Daegu semi-final, when she bumped into the English athlete Jenny Meadows at the Diamond League in Zurich. In the Daegu semi-final that Yuliya won, Meadows had been expected to go through but was over-taken for second place by the American Maggie Vessey close to the finish line. A fraction of a second, but enough to deny her a place in the final. Meadows was the fastest loser. In Zurich Yuliya spotted Meadows and saw her pain and even though her English was close to non-existent, Yuliya found a way to tell Meadows how sorry she was that Meadows hadn't made the Daegu final. Although Meadows later mistakenly recalled the exchange as having taken place in Daegu, she would be correct in saying that she sensed some guilt underlying Yuliya's expression of sympathy.

It was not the case that Yuliya was ready to abandon the Russian way. On the contrary, she spoke to Portugalov and intimated she would like more. A little more of everything. She would like better attention, better drugs, better monitoring. Please. Portugalov was non-committal. And it infuriated her. It seemed a serf would always be a serf until she could buy her freedom. She got that. But Yuliya had the money to push upwards yet he was playing some game with her. Her future was in his hands and he was deliberating.

'Don't worry, Yuliya. For London you will be ready. All other things may wait.'

So she worried more. Wait? Was she designated to finish in the group in London while Savinova had been chosen to win? It was depressing to know that she was doing everything in her powers to become a winner, only to discover that there were secret rooms she had known nothing about.

Vitaly held his tongue, realising Yuliya must feel some of what a clean athlete felt when a Yuliya or a Savinova finished ahead of them. This was a Russian version of that feeling. Yuliya was on the Russian side of the fence and the unfairness that nagged her was knowing that other athletes cheated more and cheated better. She felt frustrated, like a person who had celebrated the 50 per cent pay rise they had worked hard for, only to discover that a colleague had got a 75 per cent rise without asking. She had got what she asked for but it really galled her to find out that somebody else had got more. She felt foolish. She wasn't, after all, an exotic butterfly being observed carefully in a bell-jar but just a small part of Portugalov's broad customer base.

Portugalov, in truth, had delivered just what he had said he would. He had broken no guarantees. She got the right drugs.

She had the testing threat neutralised. She had competed 'dirty' at the 2011 Russian Indoors and would do so again at the 2012 meet. As instructed, she had texted her sample numbers to Portugalov, who passed the details to the laboratory. On 17 February 2011 she texted the sample number, 2573960. She held on to her page of the doping control forms and the magic worked. Sample number 2573960 was never heard of again. Instead, sample number 2673502 was duly filed by the Moscow laboratory into ADAMS (the Anti-Doping Administration and Management System, which co-ordinated anti-doping activities worldwide under the World Anti-Doping Code) as a negative: *Yuliya Stepanova. Officially clean.* She had done these things with the full knowledge and authorisation of ARAF's head running coach, Aleksei Melnikov, and Portugalov. That was what her money had bought her. They had never promised more. And yet the men who ran the secret pharmacy determined not just where Russians would finish against their rivals from the rest of the world, but also which Russians would finish ahead of other Russians.

Special lanes, special privileges, special means. All Portugalov's athletes were equal, but some were more equal than others. Being more equal was going to cost more money.

Chapter 19

In October 2011, Vitaly and Yuliya travelled to the US for a holiday after a difficult year. America always invigorated Vitaly. In their absence, a former Rusada colleague of Vitaly's, Alexey Slautin, found work with SOOC, the organising committee of the 2014 Winter Olympic Games, to be held in the beach-resort city of Sochi.

There was much excitement about the Games – or, as Vitaly saw the event, the latest distraction on offer from the state's bread and circuses department. People were long accustomed to the decadent novelty of being allowed to buy salami or cheeseburgers if they could afford them. Those items had been tasty at first but, all in all, less fulfilling than people had imagined. The Sochi project would show the world that Russia could afford to present a glorious theatre of dancing white elephants if it so wished. The show might grease the palms of the cronies who had sprung forth to replace the Communist Party in the new Russia but it would also gladden the souls of the down-at-heel proletariat.

Slautin hadn't been purged from his old job. He had left Rusada of his own will. Now he was to be a manager in the anti-doping department for Sochi. Not the boss of all bosses but a highly ranked individual with some influence. When his new employers sought one or two more individuals to further flesh out their staff, Slautin mentioned Vitaly's name as a good man with Olympic experience. Vitaly entered employment with SOCOG in early November 2011. Slautin's boss was Evgeny Antilsky, a man dulled by the complacency of the state employee. The workload of the anti-doping department fell on the shoulders of others.

If the Games were to demonstrate the rude well-being of Putin's Russia, many things had to be built, to work well and to be conspicuously impressive. The anti-doping department was not numbered among those things. In Sochi, the great Russian athlete would compete in an environment where the stress of worrying about positive tests had been entirely removed.[1] Behind the glorious facade, there would be some private business the world wouldn't see.

They worked minimum twelve-hour shifts, often just moving mountains of paperwork between the rival interests within the organising committee. Or composing long follow-up emails about said mountains. Vitaly's contract restricted his remuneration to eight hours' worth of pay for any given day. He found himself offering the extra time he worked as a donation towards the big show. He was dispirited by his own watery patriotism.

Commercially, of course, the usual cohorts were in charge. Construction for the Games was a brimming trough from which many slurped. Arenas, roads, railways, power plants, hotels. The final bill would top $51 billion. Global television companies would pay colossal fees to beam shots of benign palm trees growing by the Black Sea. Sponsors would flock. Tourists would gaze in wonder. This Sochi, this place was what the new nation, President Putin's Russia, was all about.

Physically Sochi bore no comparison to places like Chelyabinsk or Kursk but spiritually the Games were a snapshot of something very Russian. It is true to say there was optimism in the air. 'The best Games are created by the best people' was the slogan and many of those recruited by Sochi bought into that. For Vitaly, the difficulty was that he'd seen all this during the early days at Rusada. Now, as back then, the foot soldiers were expected to work long days with no overtime. And if you knew how the system worked, you could see that everything wasn't as it seemed. Nobody who came to Sochi seemed to notice the FSB officers who were lurking in the background, some not even in the background. What a triumph of marketing they were. Had they still been known as the KGB, their presence would not have gone unnoticed.

At one point it was agreed that Jeremy Luke, who had been in charge of the anti-doping department in Vancouver, would do some oversight to ensure that all matters anti-doping at the Sochi laboratory were in line with precedent and standards. The IOC insisted on Luke's presence. SOCOG paid for it.

There was a meeting in late 2011 where SOCOG had to explain to Luke what they had done so far. Basic information. What types of doping control stations there would be. How many doping control stations they were planning to have at various sites. How many cars would be made available. How they were going to transfer samples from the doping control stations to the lab. How long that would take. Simple logistics. At the meeting Rusada was represented in the familiar forms of Nikita Kamaev and Igor Zagorskiy. The director of the Moscow lab, Dr Rodchenkov, was also present.

Jeremy Luke was very polite and never asked anything out of line. He posed some straightforward questions and he received some short answers. He shook hands with everybody and left. The day after Luke's departure Slautin showed Vitaly a letter from the Ministry of Sports to SOCOG. The letter was bitter and plaintive. For Russia to be asked to endure the impertinence of a so-called expert from Canada? It was offensive. This expert who comes and asks these uncomfortable questions about financing for anti-doping laboratories? The cheek. The

Ministry said the relationship was not going to work and would have to be discontinued.

Luke had been approved by the IOC, however, and his visits could not be prohibited. There would be a Russian solution to this Canadian problem. All personnel smiled whenever Luke was around. Then they just worked around him. This was a glorious project, after all. Tired of the expense of keeping one step ahead of the doping police through science, Russia was going to eliminate science by performing what the Americans would call the old switcheroo.

It took just three months for Vitaly to be overwhelmed by his own misgivings. He could just keep taking the pay cheques or he could get the hell out. He tendered his resignation in January.

Vitaly had been emailing WADA since 2010. It was now early 2012 and the bulletins were stacking up. But to what end? Vitaly wasn't sure. Stuart Kemp was still his point of contact and, although the correspondence was two-way, Kemp's responses tended to be polite and matter of fact:

> 'Thanks for your note message received I will write you a longer note early next week from a new email. Regards.'

Vitaly no longer told Yuliya about the emails because talking about their mutual problem didn't help. Kemp seemed interested and sympathetic but Vitaly was hoping for more. He sensed Kemp was talking to WADA investigator Jack Robertson but he wasn't sure if people higher up at WADA were being briefed. Through the course of multiple emails, Kemp never mentioned the agency's president, John Fahey, Director General David Howman or General Counsel Olivier Niggli.

In an email on 3 August 2011 Vitaly said he'd stopped telling Yuliya about their contact because she didn't understand. He then admitted to misgivings of his own.

'And well I really don't understand myself why I keep doing it, besides that it is a right thing to do. But who does the right things nowadays?'

Vitaly was crying out for WADA to tell him what he was doing was important. To come up with a plan. To reassure him that the cheats were going to get caught. Or, if all that was impossible, just to say they believed him.

Then, on 29 February 2012, an uncommonly expansive email from Kemp arrived. Hallelujah!

'I wanted to touch base regarding the information you've given me in the past regarding your wife's preparation. You've mentioned ARAF [All-Russia Athletics Federation] are aware of tests in advance and the athletes are told in advance. Can you speculate on how ARAF would have this information?

'Finally, could you provide more details on your wife's preparation? What is she taking, how much and when? Are there specific plans over the coming months? Any details you can provide would be helpful. Regards.'

That last paragraph caused Vitaly a shiver of agitation. In most of their previous correspondence, Kemp simply responded to what Vitaly had written. It was rare for him to ask for anything specific. So why did WADA now want the minutiae of Yuliya's doping? And why not speak to him about their sudden interest in his wife?

From the moment Vitaly had first started speaking to WADA he'd resolved to be truthful. However difficult it got, he would stick to that. He had outlined the nature of the doping conspiracy in Russia for them. How it worked. Who it involved. Every elite athlete, he told them, was part of the system. To not discuss his wife's doping would have been a lie. He couldn't do that.

The irony was that the athlete they now seemed particularly interested in was Yuliya. Why? The question was obvious. The answer less so.

Ten days later Vitaly replied to Kemp. First, he tried to explain how Russian athletes, with the help of their coaches, could control when they were tested. They took their doping products, calculated the clearance time and agreed to a test after that date. The largest country in the world, with its very diverse topography, offered a natural habitat for the cheat. The IAAF sent a request to Rusada, for example, asking that a specified list of athletes be tested. Rusada got in touch with the national coach, Melnikov, and they then decided when each of those athletes would be tested. If the IAAF wanted a particular athlete tested at a particular time, they could be easily fobbed off.

'Sorry, that athlete lives in a closed city. Not possible to go there. We can get clearance but it will take more time.'

'Sorry, this athlete is at a training camp in a place so remote it would take a flight from Moscow, then another flight to a nearby city, and maybe for the last part of the journey it would be necessary to travel on a snowmobile. And then huskies or reindeer might be needed.'

The places athletes named on their whereabouts form weren't easily accessible. The athletes never went there. The doping control officers couldn't get there. All good. If, on the off chance, a tester showed up at the wrong place and at the wrong time, no one should panic. Most of Rusada's testers knew when to look the other way. If an uncooperative, non-Rusada tester showed up unannounced, the athlete had clean urine stored in the fridge for that kind of occasion.

To keep everyone happy, Russia offered up a regular supply of positives comprising those poor sacrificial lambs who weren't part of Melnikov's elite circle. Vulnerable souls not good enough to make the national team but a perfect serving to sate the need for some positive tests from Russia. Another four positives from Russia last month! Jolly good show, chaps! At least someone is catching the infernal cheats!

Vitaly knew all about this charade and much more. So WADA restricting its curiosity to questions about Yuliya's doping regimen irked him. Still, he couldn't arbitrarily halt a process that he himself had initiated. He couldn't suddenly switch to an à la carte truth menu. In an email to Kemp, he gave them what they wanted.

> 'April, for three weeks – steroids that are detectable for thirty days.'
>
> 'Late May, same steroids or lighter for three weeks.'
>
> 'Steroids come from Argentina.'
>
> 'Close to National Championships (end of June) EPO injections.'
>
> 'After National Championships (end of June), testosterone injections.'
>
> 'Close to Olympics but not in London, testosterone gel.'

Towards the end of what was a long email, Vitaly also wrote about a shift in Portugalov's attitude towards Yuliya. She'd been trying to contact him for two weeks but he wasn't responding. Finally, Portugalov had sent a text, saying that he changed his job. It was a lie. Vitaly didn't know what had changed but something had. He had the impression that Melnikov and the race-walking coach Viktor Chegin were spooked by his presence. Almost afraid of him. This in turn spooked Vitaly. He explained this to Kemp and said he felt he was getting into serious stuff. One of his final thoughts showed he wasn't entirely sure about WADA any more.

'Hmm ... and well I still hope that you are using the information for the right reasons.'

The strange story of WADA and International Doping Tests and Management (IDTM's) Ekaterina Antilskaya – Part One

Weeks later, Melnikov told coach Mokhnev that WADA had instructed the Swedish testing agency IDTM to test Yuliya. This would be a 'no notice' test that Melnikov had, of course, learned about in advance. Everybody had enough time to make sure Yuliya was properly prepared, all performance-enhancing drugs rinsed from her system. It wasn't difficult to manage. Knowing roughly when the test would happen, Yuliya listed Saranpaul on her whereabouts form in WADA's system. Saranpaul is a small, isolated town a thousand miles east of Moscow. A flight to Syktyvkar, followed by a helicopter to somewhere close, and from there a reindeer-driven sled through the snow to Saranpaul. Not a good commute for a Moscow-based DCO.

Melnikov called Yuliya with an update in early May. As well as a blood test for her biological passport, WADA wanted a urine sample for an EPO test. This was inconvenient because it meant Yuliya would have to be completely free of EPO for the test. Her EPO injections were due to clear her system sometime between 21 and 25 May. From what Melnikov was hearing, WADA was pressuring the IDTM people to get this test done, so he arranged for Yuliya to be at her mother's apartment in Kursk on 24 May, where this 'no notice' test could be carried out.

Vitaly didn't tell Yuliya he suspected the information he'd passed on to WADA was the reason she was being tested. He wanted them to test athletes, his wife included, but something about this bothered him. Was Yuliya's name one on a list of

athletes sent to IDTM or was she the only one? For almost a
year and a half Vitaly had told them everything he knew. In
return they had told him virtually nothing. He wasn't sure they
believed his story or even if they wanted to believe it. He didn't
know if they trusted him. When it came right down to it, he
didn't think they were really listening to him. Plenty of times
he'd advised them that the athletes Russia wanted to protect
could not be properly tested in their home country. WADA
half-listened. They knew enough not to trust Rusada but
not enough to realise that IDTM was no better. Instead, they
thought the Swedish-based operation would get the job done.
They were Swedes, after all. Volvos. Ikea. Abba. Safe.

Part of Vitaly felt like laughing at the waste of money. The
other part wondered why WADA didn't ask him about IDTM's
operation in Russia. Vitaly had met IDTM's woman in Moscow,
Ekaterina Antilskaya. They'd once collected samples at the same
venue. He knew exactly how Antilskaya went about things.
For starters, she enjoyed a good working relationship with
Melnikov, which meant she wasn't on the side of clean athletes.
She told him whom she needed to test, he helped to arrange
it. For Melnikov, the payback was that he determined *when* his
athletes were tested.

Vitaly and Yuliya were in Kursk on the evening of 23 May,
expecting Ekaterina Antilskaya to turn up the following day to
carry out her unannounced test. Around 8 p.m. the phone rang.
It was Antilskaya, who apologised for contacting Yuliya directly
but she'd been trying Melnikov and he wasn't picking up.

'Sorry about this,' Antilskaya said, 'but I can't get to Kursk for
tomorrow's test. Could you get to Moscow for early tomorrow
morning, say 8 a.m. ?'

'Okay.'

'One other thing. Don't change your whereabouts. Leave it
at Kursk.'

Vitaly and Yuliya set off on the late-night drive of 350 miles. At 8 a.m. at the Olimpiyskiy Sports Complex in Moscow Yuliya met Antilskaya. They did a blood test. Then Antilskaya accompanied Yuliya to a toilet, not because she wanted to watch the delivery of the urine sample but because Yuliya didn't know the way. Antilskaya stood outside the cubicle while Yuliya did what she had to do and listened to Antilskaya tell her WADA were really pushing for Yuliya to be tested. They had actually wanted poor Antilskaya to go to that out-of-the-way place beyond all the plains and the forests and the mountains, the place named in Yuliya's whereabouts form. She'd told them the second part of the journey to Saranpaul could only be taken by helicopter. Only then did they nix the idea.

Test completed, Yuliya signed the doping control form. *Location: Kursk. Time: between 10 p.m. and 11 p.m.*

'Don't worry about the time we've put on the form,' said Antilskaya, 'I will keep the sample safely in my fridge for the next fourteen hours.'

A lot of people knew how Antilskaya operated. Recording the test as having been carried out in Kursk, she would invoice IDTM for her travel and overnight expenses. IDTM would in turn invoice WADA, who would get some very clean blood and urine in return. Everyone would have a slice of the cake.

Three weeks later, Vitaly emailed Kemp with a detailed account of the bogus test carried out by IDTM. He didn't spare Antilskaya. IDTM's Moscow representative was part of Russia's doping system. Vitaly imagined this would be the end of Antilskaya's relationship with IDTM, maybe even the end of WADA's collaboration with IDTM. But if there were repercussions, no one told Vitaly.

Weeks passed, during which Yuliya regularly asked how her husband's job-hunting was progressing. Vitaly emailed Stacy Spletzer at WADA, Rob Koehler too, but there were no openings for an out-of-work anti-doping officer from Russia. Thinking that maybe IDTM would soon need a new manager in Moscow, he got in touch with the company's marketing manager, who passed his application and CV on to Denis Pioline, Head of Recruitment. In a courteous reply, Pioline said he would pass on Vitaly's details to IDTM's manager in Moscow, Ekaterina Antilskaya, who would be in touch with him. Vitaly doubted that she would. As much as he knew her modus operandi, she knew his. She never did get in touch with Vitaly.

~

Vitaly's work situation was only a little troubling to him. He appeared to critics, such as his parents in Chelyabinsk, to have become quite selective about applying the 'never quit' vow he had made for himself when he moved from Chelyabinsk to Moscow. Vitaly never saw himself as more spiritually pure than anybody else. Maybe Americans could afford such luxuries but nobody in Russia could. He paid the bribes to the traffic police when they held out their hands. He used connections and influence just like every Russian did to make life better or to stop life being worse. He had made calls and paid money to avoid a drafting request from the army when applying for the new passport he'd needed to go to the Beijing Olympics. This was life. But sport was the great escape from all that. Running, jumping, throwing, kicking, all these things were free to every Russian. That was the glory. The biggest land on the planet to play in. So why stain it with politics and corporates and corruption? Sport was different. Sport and love. And if he was odd about it? Well, a man was entitled to one or two pure passions on this earth.

In the meantime, those who knew him awaited the next big enthusiasm in his life.

For now, his main enthusiasm continued to be Yuliya. She affected him like the weather or the quality of the air or food.

Her moods affected his. Every day she continued to share a part of her life with him. He hoped that someday she might share all of her life with him. She had a quality that drew men towards her, almost as if they wanted to be bent around her little finger. Vitaly's obstinance meant he wasn't up for that trip. With her doping he always made it clear that he hated the offence but that it was his fate to love the offender.

Yuliya had performed well in 2011, and inexorably the girl from Kursk who had watched the Sydney Olympics in awe twelve years earlier was closing in on the 2012 Games in London. It was a journey that Vitaly wanted to share with her. This dream illuminated her like nothing else. When he thought about her and how close she was getting, he worried a little that the adventure could either bring them both happiness or drive them apart. It was a risk to be taken, though. No question. They would work towards it together. Now that he no longer worked for Rusada, the idea that he was a secret agent for WADA felt like a figment of his imagination, something from a hazy past life. He kept the emails going and it seemed to him they replied mostly out of courtesy.

Instead, he offered himself to Yuliya as a volunteer. He would be her personal rabbit, her pacemaker. It worked well. He was a decent runner and it was difficult to find good runners willing to sacrifice themselves day in and day out to make the pace for another. Vitaly threw himself into the grind, filling his days with the two things he loved: Yuliya and running. She seemed happy to have him around, and this was the best time they had known in their married life. They had moved past tolerating each other. They shared something now. The harder they worked, the more he liked it and the more Yuliya seemed to appreciate him.

They did interval sessions once every three or four days, maybe twenty or thirty different interval workouts: 200 metres,

300s, 400s, all mixed. Three, four or five sets. At the beginning of the season they might start with maybe fifteen times 400 metres at seventy-five seconds each, and then gradually change from fifteen times to ten times but at seventy seconds. Then go to eight times at sixty-eight seconds until they ended up doing three or four 400s at or just under sixty seconds.

There were times towards the end of the season when Yuliya was in shape to run under two minutes and by then Vitaly had become like Drew, the defeated guitarist in the duelling banjos scene from *Deliverance*. He just couldn't keep up any more. Running four 400s each in sixty seconds with 150-second recoveries in between, she might follow him for 300 metres and then leave him for dust. He would have that little extra time for recovery to be ready when she wanted to go again. He needed every second. He would catch his breath as his wife ran and he would watch her. Working together like this was perfect. She was beautiful but especially so when she ran. As if this was why she had been created. If he was compromising one belief, it was for a better belief: what this woman could be.

His email relationship with WADA continued and, though it was unfulfilling, he was committed to it. He was no longer employed by Rusada or SOCOG – a bigger concern for WADA than the state of his marriage to Yuliya – but at least he was able to paint a detailed picture of Russian sport at a micro level.

'Case Study. Name: Yuliya Rusanova. Target: London Olympics 2012.[2] Description: To show how a Russian prepares for the Olympic Games and the perceived need for performance-enhancing drugs.'

He sent emails to WADA in the evening and worked with Yuliya in the day. Did he see himself as betraying her? No more than she saw herself as betraying him. She'd always been open about her doping. He never said he wasn't writing to WADA. They got along by not talking about it. He didn't kid himself that she secretly admired what he was doing. He saw her as a victim of the system, a talent that would for ever be unfulfilled and always unhappy doing things the way she was doing them. He loved her but he didn't own her. She thought him naive, painfully simplistic. Sending his emails to WADA! Well, where was the cavalry they promised him? In its own Russian way, it all made some sort of sense.

At the Russian Indoors on 23 February 2012 Yuliya took second place. The result meant she travelled to the World Indoors in Istanbul in March. There, however, she experienced the nightmare scenario again. She put her foot on the gas and nothing happened. In her heat she had beaten the 2008 Olympic champion, but in the final she trailed home in last place. Heartbroken again.

But darker clouds were gathering. The previous month, after her silver at the National Indoor Championships and just before Istanbul, Yuliya had sent a text message to Portugalov with her sample number. She was running dirty again and he was paid to disguise it. The test was duly covered up but Yuliya had also wanted to see Portugalov to talk to him about her preparation for Istanbul. He ducked her for a few days until ten or so text messages later he sent a reply.

'Sorry, I can't help you any more.'

He had changed job, he said. Nothing else.

She didn't believe him. A guy like Portugalov whose entire life was wrapped up in helping Russian athletes do great things for the country? He doesn't walk away. Why would he? In Olympic year? Yuliya felt like the little girl she used to be, on the stairs in the house in the woods, sensing there might be wolves out there. She was powerless. Whether he was lying or not didn't matter. The text ended her working relationship with him. It was no surprise to learn later that he was still doing the same job. For some reason, she was the problem.

Vitaly heard that Portugalov was now being pressured by Russian drug control officers, the narcotics people. That was serious stuff. Distribution of steroids was a criminal offence in Russia, and it was rumoured that a criminal gang conducted its own trade in Moscow. Portugalov, though, was essential to the entire project of state-sponsored doping. That made him bulletproof. Surely. Vitaly wouldn't normally put much store by such Moscow gossip, but something was stirring.

Much later Vitaly would wonder if WADA, bound by their own endless red tape, had mentioned his name to someone in Russia. He had no proof that anyone had, but the climate changed. He recalled the moment from the summer of 2011 when Portugalov, who had previously been okay with him, had started to cut him dead.

Meanwhile, Yuliya returned from Istanbul deeply disheartened. In two World Championship finals she'd pulled two last places. She felt faith in her was ebbing away. Russia's pool of 800 metres women was deep and talented. It would be easy to wake up one day with a great future behind you. She decided to prove them wrong. She would train harder than ever. She was going to go to London 2012. She would make the final there. There would be no last place. The dream didn't end that way.

Training camps were the same as the year before. They went to Portugal again. The same as last year, except for the names they used when checking into their hotel. They pretended to be different Russians from the Russians they really were. Just in case the testers came.

In the sunshine Yuliya worked hard and well. It was early April, with a lot of heavy grind work needed, but Vitaly could see that she was already in under-two-minute form. London loomed once more on the horizon.

During the training camp Melnikov took some time out to speak quietly with Yuliya. First of all, Russia. The problem with dear Mother Russia was that she did not need athletes who lagged home last in major finals. Mother Russia didn't send her athletes to major finals so they could know the joy of taking part. When your country said 'come forth' it didn't mean 'come fourth'. Or worse. Mother Russia was disappointed in Yuliya, but Yuliya would get one more chance and the Federation would prepare her in the Federation's own way for the National Championships.

Having delivered the message from Mother Russia, Melnikov finally reassured Yuliya that she would again be able to run dirty at the Nationals. If everything went well until then. The only way ARAF could create the outcome where the preferred athletes qualified was by letting them compete dirty at the Nationals. That way the cream would rise to the top. Melnikov felt it was only right to put Yuliya in the picture.

'And Mr Portugalov?' she asked.

'No need to worry. He is well and he is preparing a lot of medal-contenders for the Olympics. Just not you, Yuliya.'

The official position was that there were two problems from Portugalov's perspective. He no longer believed that Yuliya could win a medal at a major championship because, sad to say, she was not strong enough psychologically. Also, frankly, he was spooked by Yuliya's husband. Had someone warned Portugalov that Vitaly was talking to WADA or to the IAAF? Very sad. In the old days informants did these despicable things for a few kopeks or through fear. Now this? Melnikov himself didn't know whether or not Vitaly was informing. It all seemed like such a strange state of affairs that he thought it wise not to speculate. He would say, though, that he didn't like Vitaly being around training. Nothing personal. He just didn't enjoy his presence.

As a sign of his good faith, Melnikov proposed that he would go to Portugalov back in Moscow and intercede on Yuliya's behalf. What was there to lose?

Yuliya was beginning to think there might be a lot to lose. In the Algarve, in the long amber evenings, the athletes and their coaches gossiped and talked shop. They were explicit about the options Portugalov offered on the magic-carpet ride to success. 'First class plus' cost $5,000 straight up plus 5 per cent from all prize money. Yuliya was getting by in economy for $1,000 plus 5 per cent for a season. And she was finishing last in major finals. Perhaps the problem wasn't her psychological make-up or who she had married. She wasn't being prepared for anything more than she was achieving.

Right after the World Indoor Championships in Istanbul in March, Yuliya underwent an out-of-competition test conducted by Rusada. Melnikov spoke to her about it. He was apologetic, saying it should not have happened. A ghost in the machine. A gremlin in the system. It was very disappointing. The Federation and Rusada had an agreement in place not to test athletes who might be in the International Registered Testing Pool during that period of time. If it was any consolation, the same thing had happened to the great Mariya Savinova. Twice. It was not good. Nobody was happy. Heads would roll. Yuliya paid little attention. If it had really happened to Savinova (twice), for the amount of money she was paying Portugalov, the problem would have been dealt with.

In the meantime, Yuliya was more worried about her body. She had pulled something high in her right leg while at the Portuguese training camp. Nothing major, just a strong tweak. She dismissed it as no big deal. She would work through it. At some point soon she would take a rest for a few days. It was Olympic year. No matter what anybody else thought, she was psychologically strong.

They went to Kursk for a few days and she kept on training. Then it was eastwards to Kyrgyzstan to yet another training camp, in the thin air at Lake Issyk-Kul. For another four or five days the leg hurt, but she kept training, pushing and pushing. This was no time to show weakness. Then one day she just couldn't run any more. It was the middle of April, and London was a little more than three months distant.

They did an MRI. Cold science brought bad news. The picture told its story. The 2012 Olympics would just be another television show for Yuliya. And suddenly she was once again difficult to be around. Vitaly could understand that. What he didn't understand was the lingering influence of Mokhnev.

Vitaly had known about Mokhnev's relationship with Yuliya before he met the man, so there was always a strain there. Now, though, Mokhnev could not accept that his erstwhile protégé would not be competing in London. He had put years of investment into this project and now his glory had been stolen. Who was to blame for this? He knew who. Mokhnev felt Vitaly was to blame. Yuliya, his girl, running with an enthusiastic amateur as a rabbit? Who had heard of such foolishness? She had nobody to check her stretches, her warm-ups and her warm-downs. What could be expected of such a harum-scarum arrangement?

As the Russian National Championships approached, Mokhnev's bitterness ate at him like a cancer. If Yuliya didn't compete at the Nationals, that was the end of the Olympic dream. His calls and his pressure increased. But the injury wasn't responding to treatment. The only sensible decision was not to run. Mokhnev couldn't bring himself to make that decision.

Vitaly and Yuliya decided there was only one way to get some peace. They would leave Kursk for a while and go to Vitaly's home in Chelyabinsk. Being away from Kursk would take the pressure off. Disappointment had broken Yuliya. Mokhnev's calls weren't helping. In Chelyabinsk Vitaly couldn't heal

Yuliya's injury but he could put her mind back in the right place. He persuaded her to look to the future and not to the past. They would go to America in the summer and there they could avoid seeing most of the London Olympics. When they returned, things would be different. They had many talks about her future as an athlete. A part of Yuliya's life had ended but she was Russian and conditioned to the possibility of disappointment.

'Look,' he said, 'for most athletes and people from many other Olympic sports, life happens in four-year cycles. This four-year cycle just ended for you with nothing. We should start right now making changes for the next four-year cycle. That's the only response.'

She agreed with him. He continued a little more boldly.

'Maybe we should start with your coach. Are you going to have Mokhnev around for another four years? Doing the same shit? Giving you the same pressures? He's not a coach for an elite athlete. You know that.'

Again she agreed.

'So who is the best? If you were to change coaches, who would you choose?'

One name rose above all others: Vladimir Kazarin. Kazarin had been Mariya Savinova's coach. Over the previous two years Savinova hadn't lost a single major competition. European Championships, Indoor, Outdoor. World Championships, Indoor, Outdoor. Everything was hers and she was a sure thing to win at the London Olympics. She got the best attention from Portugalov but she got the best coaching from Kazarin too. Vitaly and Yuliya spoke to athletics people in Chelyabinsk. They all shared the same high opinion of Kazarin. The job was his if he chose to accept it.

On the long drive from Chelyabinsk back to Moscow, they were excited. Vitaly had an idea. Why wait? Many athletes were in Cheboksary in camps, getting ready for the Nationals there in a few weeks. Vitaly rang his dad, who had some contact with coaches back in Chelyabinsk. Could he get a mobile number for Kazarin quickly? Done. Yuliya dialled the number.

'Hello? I am Yuliya Rusanova. I am an 800 metres runner—'

Kazarin interrupted to say that of course he knew of her and what she did. She asked if they could meet in the near future to talk.

'Okay,' he said.

'Where are you?'

'I am in Cheboksary training my athletes.'

'Well,' said Yuliya, 'if you want, I could come to you in a few hours.'

'Okay,' he said, realising that this woman meant business.

In Cheboksary Yuliya told him she was thinking about a change of coach. Could he take her on? She worked hard. She had potential. Surely he could see that? In the next four years she would be coming into her prime as a runner. He said only that the National Championships were to be held in a few weeks' time so she should come along to those. Everyone would be there – head coach Melnikov, Dr Portugalov, all the top officials. They could discuss it in more detail then but, in general, he said he was interested.

Vitaly sat in his car while Yuliya met with Kazarin. While they were talking, Vitaly saw Savinova and her husband leaving the training camp. There was a locked gate that had to be opened especially for them. Their black Maserati slowed and out of the car stepped Savinova to open the gate. Savinova. A Maserati. Kazarin. It was a sign that these things seemed linked. By the time Yuliya got back to the car, Vitaly felt as optimistic as she did. As they drove back to Moscow they were the happiest they had been since before the injury.

Chapter 20

Cheboksary three weeks later. National Championships

Yuliya was speaking to Kazarin in a car parked maybe twenty metres away. Vitaly sat and waited in his own car. He knew his presence made hardcore athletics people uneasy. He was still the fox in their little henhouse. He didn't need to startle anybody today. *Nobody here but you chickens*, he thought. After twenty minutes Yuliya came back. She was crying. Kazarin had consulted with Portugalov and with Melnikov. They had advised him not to touch her with a barge pole.

'He said that they told him I have blood passport problems.'

'But everybody has blood passport problems. Since February. That's the rumour. Kazarin knows that. Nobody talks about anything else.'

'And he said my husband is also a problem.'

'Did he?'

'Yes, he said that. Vitaly, you are ruining my fucking life.'

He had no real argument. He *was* ruining her life. What she believed impacted him in marginal ways. What he believed was crushing her. When she calmed down he asked her a question.

'Is that it then? No hope?'

He was talking about Kazarin, not about their marriage.

'He told me that he was saying no, but he said to call him again after the Olympics. Maybe he will talk to them again.'

It was not an easy evening. When a wife tells her husband that he is ruining her life and he agrees with her, it is not a time for a candlelit dinner.

In the morning they drove home from Cheboksary. Silence filled the car. Vitaly weighed up the situation. Anti-doping wasn't even part of his life now except for exchanging emails with WADA. Well, not exactly exchanging. He would write and WADA would acknowledge that he had written. It was not dialogue. He felt rebuffed everywhere. Yuliya never asked him what he was writing to WADA. It was of no interest to her. Did she care about how honest he was in his emails? Or did she know and just dismiss it all as foolishness?

Two days passed and things got better between them. They went ahead with the trip to America. Blue skies. Clean light. Friendly faces. Vitaly showed Yuliya the America that he considered to be his own America, the place he knew and loved.

When Vitaly was in eighth grade, his mother asked him one day out of the blue if he would like to study English in another country. Vitaly was thirteen. 'No, thank you,' he said.

He thought about it later and wasn't sure why he had dismissed the idea. He wanted to see the world beyond Chelyabinsk. A year later the issue came up again. This time he said yes as if it was the last hope of saving his life.

'England or America?' his mother asked.

He was a fan of American sports. He followed the score-cards in the Russian weekly *Sport Express*. The biggest cars were American.

'America,' said Vitaly.

The Stepanovs had been told that Vitaly would go to private school not far away from New York City. A place called New Jersey. He ended up in Pennsylvania. Allentown. In Russia you arrange for one thing and you get something different. You deal with it. He fell back on sports. A kid called Jared Markowitz asked him to come out to soccer one day. Vitaly went, played a game and then for days afterwards his muscles ached and he walked stiffly.

'You are fifteen and after one soccer game you walk like an old man?' he scolded himself.

So from then on, he did every sport he could. One day, after months of nodding at each other, Jared looked at Vitaly and noted a solemnity he hadn't seen before.

'Hey, Vitaly, you don't look so happy today. You always look so happy.'

Vitaly was embarrassed that he lacked sufficient English to discuss this. So he said the first funny thing he could think of.

'Oh. Yes, my mother died.'

Jared's face twisted with pain and embarrassment. Uh–oh.

'Joke,' said Vitaly. 'It is a joke. She did not die. Ha!'

Jared and Vitaly were tight after that.

When Vitaly had been in America for almost a year, his family had come west to take a look at his world. They hired a rental car and just drove. For Russians, this America felt small and cosy. They drove the 500 miles from Philadelphia to Toronto and then looped back to Niagara Falls. Then they pointed the car south again for a 1,300-mile jaunt to Orlando, Florida. They'd rented a gorgeous cherry-red Oldsmobile Model 88 that felt like the American Dream on shiny hub-capped wheels. It was late August. The air was hot and humid, but Russian kids never ask 'Are we there yet?' Vitaly was sixteen and in love with this country.

In the summer of 2012, with the Olympics Games now making other people's dreams, he took Yuliya on a trip that followed the same route the Stepanovs had taken when Vitaly was still an American schoolboy.

'And this is the site where my father tipped a man twenty

dollars for helping with jump leads. My father has never been the same since.'

They drove from Allentown to Niagara Falls down to Orlando and Disney World. They saw friends and caught up with Jared. Yuliya made an effort with her English. Friends made an effort with Yuliya. Her injury was healing. Maybe as a couple they were too.

WADA and the Stuart Kemp correspondence seemed like another life. At one stage Kemp had offered to meet with Yuliya, and Vitaly had asked him for advice on how he might broach the idea of such a meeting with his wife. Russian athletes didn't tend to have meetings with WADA reps on their to-do lists. Kemp replied that he'd discuss the matter with a colleague, and that was the last Vitaly heard of it. The idea withered and died, and the 2012 holiday in the USA was WADA-free. This was just a couple of months after the 'no notice tests' farce with IDTM. Vitaly's faith in WADA was waning slightly. Here he was in America, close to their backyard in Montreal, and they didn't think he was worth meeting, even with the added incentive of meeting an athlete who was part of the Russian system. To offer to meet and then not hear back was dispiriting. Instead, he worked on the personal and enjoyed showing Yuliya his America.

For three years they had skirmished constantly with each other. The option of a permanent split had been frequently invoked by Yuliya. There weren't a lot of people they could talk to about their problems.

'I'm Vitaly, and I'm a doping control officer. This is my wife, Yuliya, an athlete in the state doping system. Our story? Well, we got married within two months of meeting each other. It was all a bit sudden. Can you help us?'

'You are having problems? Please excuse us while we fall down and pretend to be surprised.'

When they fought, they fought like dogs in a pit. On good days they looked at each other and wondered why. The good days were rare but many of them were in America.

~

While Yuliya had sat nursing her injury, she'd watched the Russian women shape up to the challenge of the London 2012 Olympics. In the space of two 1500 metres races in June that year, eight Russian women posted times that placed them in the world top twenty for the year. Runners were dropping anything from five to twenty seconds off their best times for the previous year. In the 800 metres at the Russian National Championships in Cheboksary in early July, six of the eight finalists ran under 1:59. Russia was showing a depth of talent not seen in world athletics since the Chinese middle-distance women coached by Ma Junren in the early 1990s. Not being part of it hurt.

London 2012 was a strange beast of a sporting competition. A packed stadium all day and evening, a tumultuous atmosphere, the countries of the world at play in one of the great cities. That was how it felt at the time. Hindsight would offer a different take. The countries of the world were cheating each other. The women's 1500 metres final was to become infamous. Six of the first nine to cross the line had served or would serve bans for doping.

Yekaterina Martynova, who presumably had the protection of the authorities at doping control, had clocked a 4:02.75 in Zhukovsky in June.[1] She ran a languid 4:13.86 in a slow heat in London and failed to get past the first round. Her two compatriots had mixed fortunes. Yekaterina Kostetskaya – coached, like Martynova, by Svetlana Pleskach-Styrkina – finished ninth but later had her result scratched for doping offences.[2] The 1500 metres final was won by the Turk, Asli Cakir Alptekin, who later had her title stripped following a suspension for blood doping. Her compatriot Gamze Bulut was to be elevated from the silver to the gold but in March 2016 it was announced that Bulut was being investigated for abnormal violations in her biological passport. She received a four-year ban and her results from 2011 through to 2016 were voided.

All of this was good news for Tatyana Tomashova, who herself had been banned on the eve of the Beijing Olympics, along with six other Russian athletes, for 'a fraudulent substitution of urine which is both a prohibited method and also a form of tampering with the doping control process.' She received a two-year ban later in 2008. In London Tomashova ran a disappointing 4:10.90 in the final to finish fourth but, as both Turkish medallists had their results nullified, in 2018 Tomashova was eventually elevated to the silver-medal position.[3]

Time would also bring several amendments to the results table for the women's 800-metre final in London. All three of the Russian competitors reached the final but later received bans for doping. Elena Arzhakova finished sixth in the final but was suspended for doping in 2013.[4] In November 2015, the gold medallist Mariya Savinova and the bronze medallist Ekaterina Poistogova were among five Russian runners whom WADA recommended receive lifetime bans for doping. Following final decisions from CAS, Caster Semenya of South Africa became a gold medallist five years after the race, having finished second on the day. Despite Poistogova receiving a two-year ban backdated from October 2014, her London result was unaffected and she received a silver medal.

The London Games daily brought depressing dispatches from the world Yuliya had lived in. Distracted by the great festival of cheating, nobody noticed that at the same time Yuliya, still banned, had briefly enhanced her CV. Yevgeniya Zinurova had won the 2011 European Indoor Championships 800 metres title in Paris, in a race where Yuliya came home third. Just before the London Games she was stripped of that title, having been sanctioned for abnormal blood passport values.[5] Her gold medal from Paris was also taken away. That meant the gold now went to Jenny Meadows, who learned she was a European champion on the same day that she was left out of Great Britain's Olympic team for London. France's Linda Marguet – who had finished .8 of a second behind Yuliya – was initially bumped up from fourth place to bronze, while Yuliya (briefly) became a European Indoors silver medallist. Rather than it not being over until the fat lady sings, in athletics it ain't over until the stored samples are opened. That could be anything up to ten years later.[6]

Vitaly and Yuliya had returned to Russia during the second week of the Games, when the athletics programme commanded the world's attention. In Moscow's heat, the detente between them vanished as if controlled by a switch. It was unspoken between them but every television shot was a bitter reminder that Yuliya should have been in London. As such, every day the tension between herself and Vitaly was as heavy and stifling as the humidity.

If anything was going to save them at this point, it was to have an enemy who they could unite against. Fortunately, the Moscow apartment was being shared now with Vitaly's brother, Igor, and his girlfriend, another Olga. Too many people. Too little space. Zero patience. Bad time.

Vitaly had been sent to America when Igor was just seven years old. The brothers had never been close and they had been raised differently. Vitaly was often surprised at how frank his parents were in telling people they had decided not to make the same mistakes with Igor that they had made with Vitaly. He was presented as a failed experiment. Something they had tried but that hadn't turned out so well. Vitaly was shiftless by comparison with Igor, a dreamer and an idealist, while his brother had always been hard-working and a serious student.

They paced the apartment as if it were a cage holding two separate species. Every movement made and every word uttered seemed to irritate somebody else. The tension became so bad that Vitaly suggested selling the apartment and splitting the money, with both couples then able to just go their separate ways. Igor said the apartment wasn't theirs to sell. That it still belonged to their parents, in case Vitaly had forgotten. But Vitaly figured that if they sold a decent central Moscow apartment like this, his parents could end up owning two or perhaps three apartments a little bit further out in the suburbs. That would be acceptable as a solution, surely? The inflated price they would derive due to its location was attractive. From Chelyabinsk word came that Sergey and Elena were backing Igor. They had endured enough of Vitaly's investment advice for one lifetime. At that point, Vitaly ceased communication with all Stepanovs, and the apartment fell into a long cold war.

Vitaly now had half a marriage and no family. But time passed whether you were happy or not. That much he knew. By late August Yuliya felt her injury was healed. Savinova had won in London. Russia had excelled and, as yet, nobody was asking questions as to why they had excelled. Coach Kazarin would surely be happy. Maybe it was time to go and see him again.

They met in Moscow this time. It was the same routine. Kazarin would talk to Melnikov again and he would revisit Portugalov. If they were okay with it, he would take Yuliya on board. They were already thinking about Rio 2016. For that potential they might overlook a lot.

Days passed before Kazarin called. He would take Yuliya into his system. She would have to switch her home region from Kursk to Sverdlovsk, where Kazarin and his club were located. Yuliya said goodbye to Kursk without sentiment. This was a new life. A new chapter. Except she was still married to Vitaly Stepanov. They decided that Vitaly would no longer go to training camps. Kazarin would never have to see him. Neither would Melnikov or Portugalov. It would be as if Vitaly didn't exist. He would live in Moscow. He would look for a regular job and start working like a normal person.

'Well, you will have lots of free time,' said Yuliya. 'You will have to do something not to miss me.'

Miss her? It was hard to tell if she was being funny sometimes. Perhaps what she really meant was he would have to have something to stop him interfering with her life.

~

As Yuliya's new coach was based elsewhere, she would be running for that elsewhere place in the future. Not Kursk. Early in 2012, while she was still contracted to the Kursk region, the local authority had announced the availability of extra funds for five or six local athletes who had a shot at making the Olympic Games. Cash in the region of $900 a month for four months. The chosen few were called in and informed of their small good fortune.

'Here is your first month's money. Just sign this paper to say that you have received all the money for the four months. That saves on paperwork and you will get the money for the remaining months later on.'

They signed. They got paid for one month. The remaining money ended up in the pockets of officials. Now Yuliya needed Kursk's approval to make the transfer, but she wanted her money too. It was not a life-changing sum but she was experiencing a life-changing attitude towards being hustled.

Mr Shaev was the city's director of athletics. An unlikely sort. He was a tall, unhealthy man with flappy folds of flesh dipping down over his sweatpants and a face florid from the effort of hauling the whole heap of himself around. His look was topped with a thicket of unruly hair the colour of rust. His confederate Alexander Markovchin strove for the same effect. When he first rose to his position as Chairman of Physical Culture and Sports Committee of Kursk region, he had been lean and hungry-looking. Three years later, the pay and the perks carousel had bloated him. He had furnished his expanding face with a rakish moustache.

Yuliya went first to Shaev, who bounced her over to Markovchin, the de facto minister of sports. She went to see him in his office within the House of the Soviets on Kursk's crumbling Red Square. Markovchin bounced her back to Shaev. The game went on until it became clear that, yes, she could have the approval to transfer but, no, sadly the cash was out of the question.

She and Vitaly conferred. The lost money was annoying, but being given the runaround by two fools was worse. Vitaly made a suggestion. Yuliya returned to speak to Shaev and asked him again what had happened with the money. Shaev was bored with the game now. This little blondie from the wrong part of town was no use to Kursk any more. She was injured. She was moving away to compete elsewhere. And she was pissing him off.

'Look,' he said, 'we have a football team and they need money also. It's not all about you. You didn't even make it to London anyway.'

He was cocky. She was wrong about the money she was owed, he said. Actually it was 89,000 roubles not 36,000. He was surprised she hadn't done her sums if she was really in such need. She was dismissed. This time, though, her phone had recorded every word. Now Vitaly set off to pay a visit to Chairman Markovchin.

'So, Chairman,' said Vitaly, cutting to the chase, 'Yuliya is leaving your region but your employee is not ready to pay back all the money that you owe to Yuliya as an employee. Shaev sends Yuliya to you. You send her back. We need your help.'

Markovchin was jumpy.

'I have no idea what you are talking about.'

'Well, I have this recording of Mr Shaev. Will I play it to you?'

'Are you recording us now?'

'Does it matter? Am I? Am I not? How lucky do you feel?'

'If you are recording us right now, I am going to call security and I am going to take you out. Are you recording me now?'

Vitaly let the seconds tick by. *One . . . Two . . . Three . . .* By three Markovchin was hauling himself to his feet. *Four . . . Five . . .* By five, sweat was dripping towards his moustache. *Five and a half . . . And six.*

'No, I'm not recording you.'

Markovchin collapsed into his chair again.

'I will discuss the issue but only in the presence of my sports lawyer, the man from the Ministry.'

The sports lawyer wore a suit that said that he was badly paid. His manner wasn't any more impressive than his garb. Vitaly filled him in on the situation.

'Your guy owes Yuliya almost 90,000 roubles. We want to leave quietly. All we need is your help.'

'No, no, no,' Chairman Markovchin interjected. 'Not true. Look, let me go outside for a few minutes.'

He vanished. The lawyer filled the vacuum with an impromptu speech. Rules. Value of. Officials. Respect for. Documents. Character of.

Vitaly had a question: 'Are you getting a cut out of this? No? So why cover for them?'

Markovchin returned.

'Can I give it to them in cash right now?'

The lawyer was crestfallen. He hadn't even got to offer counsel.

'No,' he said, 'the money must come from the regional athletics organisation, not from the Ministry.'

'But I have it!' said Markovchin. 'I have the money.'

So, in order to do things right, they trooped back to Shaev's office again. Yuliya, Vitaly and the lawyer waited inside. Shaev waddled in and sulkily handed over 90,000 roubles, eighteen 5,000-rouble notes in cash to Vitaly.

Vitaly fished a 1,000-rouble note from his pocket: 'Your change.'

Yuliya admired Vitaly so much at that moment that it could even have been love she was feeling.

~

She was gone through most of September, October and November while Vitaly looked for a job. Every time she called him she sounded happy. Every conversation ended the same way, with her asking if he had found a job yet. He hadn't, but he wondered if she mightn't be looking for work soon herself. One night Kazarin, after some drinks, had fleshed out a rumour that had been circulating since spring. While everybody at the top of Russian athletics had been busy beating tests and dodging testers, they had taken their eyes off the road. The new biological passport system was an articulated truck and it was coming at them, head on.

The IAAF had introduced the passport system in 2009 as part of a radically different approach by anti-doping authorities who were weary of not being able to test for substances that very few people knew existed. The passport system approached the problem from the other side, noting fluctuations in key measurements in an athlete's body. Any spikes from the generous parameters that were deemed to be normal would cause sirens to ring. The Rodchenkovs and the Portugalovs had been complacent. Now athletes were huddling over laptops, looking up their own results on WADA's ADAMS system and trying to interpret their meaning.

The names of ninety-five Russian athletes had already come up as showing irregularities in their biological passports. Nothing was confirmed yet but everybody had an opinion. There was bubbling anger among those athletes who had been paying good money to be sheltered from such disasters. It was agreed that there was no way a country could be asked to suspend ninety-five athletes at once. That would be an outrage.

There were whispers that some athletes had already discreetly accepted 'invisible suspensions'. It was post-Olympic year, so these athletes would announce an unfortunate injury or the need for some time off and they would just vanish for a while with their dignity intact. One of Kazarin's athletes, Anna Alminova, had taken this option.[7]

Of course, medallists and hot prospects would be the last to be sacrificed as the authorities made their way down the list. By that criteria, however, dozens of athletes would be abandoned to their fate. The loss of domestic credibility to the Russian system would be immense. There was nothing for it though. They would have to herd Russian athletes towards WADA while waving the white flag and begging to at least be allowed to cut deals.

Yuliya's calls home betrayed her mounting stress. The Portugalovs and Rodchenkovs had screwed up. They had outlived their usefulness but their expiry date had come at precisely the wrong time in her career. It was going to be dog eat dog for a while.

Concern for his wife prompted Vitaly to write another email to Stuart Kemp. The problem, he explained to Kemp, was that the most important men in Russia's doping chain hadn't even understood how the athlete biological passport (ABP) system worked. Portugalov, Rodchenkov and Melnikov hadn't worked out that a clean sample in doping control was as useful to the ABP police as a dirty one. A clean sample showed the norm and, once the norm was established, it became the measure against which every other test result would be measured. If your haematocrit had always been in the 41–43 range, for example, how did you explain it now being 46? Vitaly wondered if Kemp could help. It was strongly rumoured that Yuliya was one of the ninety-five suspected positives. Kazarin had told her she'd have to choose between an official ban and an unofficial one. Was this actually the case? What Vitaly was hoping was that someone at WADA might have a look at Yuliya's ABP numbers and tell her if they were problematic. If they could do that, Yuliya would at least know what her choices were.

As for Mr Portugalov, Vitaly explained, Kazarin was reporting him to be done with tending to the chemical needs of athletes. Portugalov had made enough money and didn't need the hassle any more. And now that he himself was out of work, Vitaly thanked Kemp for passing on his job application to his colleagues at WADA. He added that he didn't want to seem too pushy, and he didn't mention he was under a lot of pressure from his wife to find work. A man needs his dignity. Vitaly had other reasons for concern. When Yuliya had begun working with Kazarin, there had been the inevitable conversation about doping.

'What have you been taking, Yuliya?'

She had reeled off a long list of substances and supplements, both legal and illegal. Kazarin had cheerfully suggested that some human growth hormone would be a help. He'd added a few new names to the list. Dehydrochloromethyltestosterone. Mestanalone. Methenolone acetate. And so on.

Vitaly had actually lost track. Yuliya's diet read like a pharma brochure. And then there were the injections. Vitaly feared the system was being criminally reckless with his wife's health.

If she was one of the ninety-five to get sanctioned, if she had to take two years off, would it really be such a bad thing?

What were the odds of it happening? She was 'officially' deemed to be promising. That was why Kazarin had taken her on.[8] Was she a protected species, though? Would her last injury make her expendable? He didn't imagine Yuliya was thinking that far ahead. He didn't think she realised how cold the big machine could be when you were no longer deemed athletically hot.

In the middle of December, Vitaly was offered a job with the hotel chain Novotel. It was a management position within an antiseptic set-up out near Sheremetyevo airport. He was surprised to learn that the post was not the lowest management position they had. They asked him to start on a Monday morning at nine. Bring the necessary documents. He woke up that morning and drove out towards the old airport. Sheremetyevo had changed since he had flown out of the dowdy single terminal to America when he was just fifteen. Gleaming terminals were being built, parking lots were shooting up, shops and chain hotels had arrived. Sheremetyevo was making more progress than Vitaly.

By the entrance to the hotel, he sat in his car. He kept the engine running and the heating switched on. Every time he tried to get out of the car something pinned him to the seat. Was this really what he wanted to do? Be a flunkey in a suit? He didn't know what he wanted to do, but this was not it.

'Look,' he said to himself, 'you were offered a job. You have been looking for work for three months and this is the best offer you have been given and the best you are going to be given. If you work hard you will be able to grow. Surely. You are good with people. The money is going to be useful.'

He texted the manager of the hotel to tell him that he had received a better offer. He wished it were true. By now Yuliya and Vitaly were in the familiar standoff, pistols drawn.

'Not being able to get a job is forgivable, Vitaly. Not even *wanting* a job though?'

He conceded and promised to act. Just before New Year he took a job as a taxi driver. He had always felt serene in the madness of Moscow traffic. The cab company was a five-minute walk from the apartment. The hours were flexible. It was all good. In theory.

When Yuliya arrived back from her Chelyabinsk training camp they had the apartment to themselves as Igor and his girlfriend had gone to Australia for a month. Vitaly had a job. It was the space they should have needed. Yet things were strained. Every evening Yuliya just started in with her unhappiness.

'I am leaving you. This doesn't work. You don't have a real job. You have nothing. You have never made me happy. You are ruining everything.'

By the turn of the year, they had decided to put themselves out of their misery. They headed to the registry office. She was right. Enough madness. Divorce would release them both. Yet, even as they pulled up at the registry office, he hoped the damned place would be closed. It was open. *Yeah, thank you, Russia*, Vitaly thought.

The man they spoke to was matter-of-fact.

'Do you have children?'

'No.'

'Good. Property?'

'No.'

'Even better.'

They filed the divorce documents in sullen silence, rebuking each other in the cursive of their signatures at the bottom of the page. Ending a marriage was like a minor medical procedure.

'This is how it works,' said the man. 'We are open today but for the next week we will be closed for the holidays. We add the days when our office is closed on to your traditional thirty-day wait. So come back to us on 8 February. Both of you may come but really only one of you needs to.'

And that would be it. No hassle. No fuss. No future. The one thing Russia did really efficiently, Vitaly thought, was the administration of misery even while everything else took an age. Soon they would each just be characters in the stories their friends told. 'What were you thinking?' their friends would say, laughing.

The holiday season was beginning. Moscow had its party clothes on. They had just signed divorce papers but instead of leaving the office and going their separate ways, they walked to their car and just sat inside. Condemned to each other for another while at least. Driving home, Yuliya spoke.

'Now that I am free, Vitaly, I can be honest with you. But I need a drink.'

So they stopped at a store and bought cheap wine.

Okay, Vitaly thought. *Enjoy your wine. Enjoy your little moment telling me whatever it is that you want to tell me. This will soon be over.*

They pulled up at the apartment. It was cold but there were holiday drunks already on the street. She drank her wine. She let the light go out and she held the coldness inside her, like a small fridge with a sealed door. He sat and watched. Braced himself.

Chapter 21

They say that it's better to be slapped in the face by the truth than to be kissed by a lie. Almost free, she slapped him again and again with her cruel truths.

'You have ruined my life, Vitaly.'

'Okay. You've said that before. Is that it?'

'No. Because of you I always have more problems. Always.'

'Okay.'

Back when she'd agreed to marry him, hadn't he wondered why? He figured she'd thought, *Yeah, Vitaly is a good person and Mokhnev will be upset. Two birds, one stone.* It hadn't worked out so perfectly.

'For the past three years since we married I have been cheating on you with Mokhnev.'

'Mokhnev? Okay. You've said it now. Happy?'

'And now I have found somebody else. I met him while I was in training camp in November and December.'

'Okay. Okay.'

'We have spoken about marriage.'

'You spoke to this person about marriage while we are still married?'

'Yes, I did. I think if I stay with you I will always cheat on you.'

'Okay.'

Three years with Mokhnev her old coach. And now somebody new. Vladimir. Another 800 metres runner.

'And guess what, Vitaly? He really listens. He understands.'

She was almost free. She had nothing to lose. The knife was turning and Vitaly absorbed it all. He was not educated. He didn't have a proper job. He was nothing but wasted years and stupid dreams. He had been writing about her to WADA. He was not a man to be married to.

Then again, Yuliya. Fuck you. I don't deserve this.

That night he loved her and hated her in equal amounts. She withdrew into angry silence before she slept. His passivity driving her mad. Vitaly's brain wouldn't switch off, crackling away for most of the night. Bad thoughts. Good thoughts. All sorts. He had stayed on his feet but she had made him bleed.

Mokhnev. For fuck's sake. He had always suspected it but he had no evidence. Perhaps he didn't want to know. At the training camps not organised by the ARAF there was never a masseuse. So the coach did the massage. Every time Yuliya went for massage, Vitaly had wondered about Mokhnev with his old-man hands all over her. There were times when he saw them fighting and he knew their fights were not the way a coach and athlete fight.

But you were my wife and I believed in you, Yuliya . . .

They even had the discussion once. He recalled it now. It was the spring of 2010 and she was in a training camp but she had come home to Moscow. They were in a Moscow park. He had seen messages on her phone and he was just screaming at her. Right there in the park.

'Why are you doing this? You are cheating on me. Why?'

She had just looked at him quietly.

'I am not cheating.'

There was no emotion. She just didn't care. She lied with iced blood, as cold as a person could get. He was in the park, screaming. People were watching. And she just said it flat and cold.

'I am not cheating on you.'

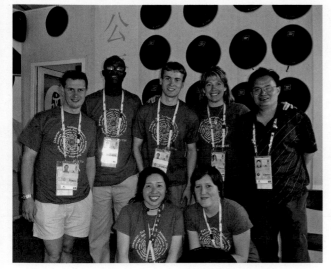

Being invited by WADA to be part of their team at the Beijing Games in 2008 was a thrill for Vitaly Stepanov, centre back. To his immediate left is Stacy Spletzer, one of his first contacts at WADA.

Seen here with WADA's Stuart Kemp and Tom May, Vitaly (left) enjoyed his trip to the 2008 Olympics. He didn't know then what he would learn over the following two years.

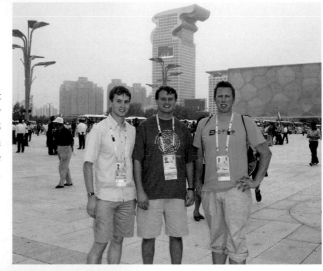

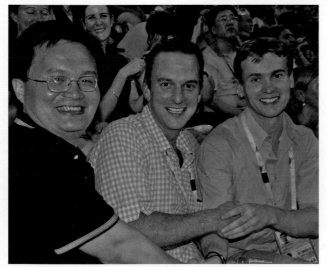

Vitaly Stepanov with Wang Xinzhai, Department Director from Chinese Sport, and USADA chief executive Travis Tygart at the 2008 Beijing Games.

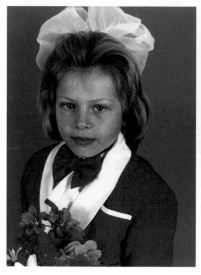

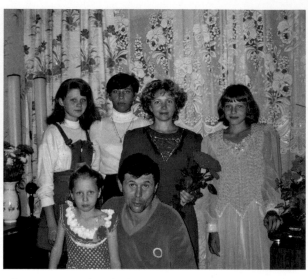

When Yuliya Rusanova was nine, a photographer came to her school and brought some fancy clothes and flowers. This was the result.

The Rusanova family; back row, from left, sister Katia, Lusya (Katia's friend), mum Lyubov, Yuliya. Front row, sister Angelina and dad Igor.

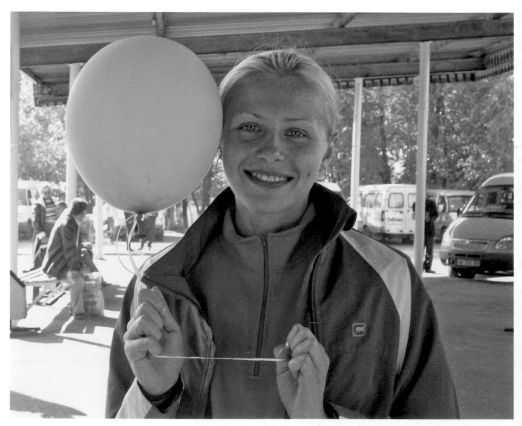

After a cross-country race in Orenburg, 21-year-old Yuliya is at the bus station ready for the journey back to Kursk. The balloon would eventually burst.

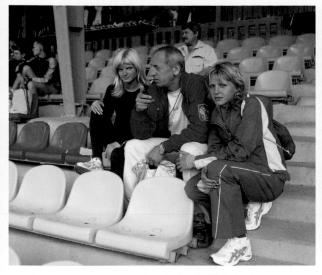

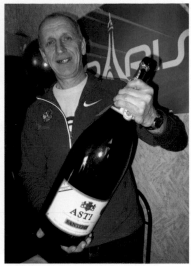

A young Yuliya (r) with her then coach Vladimir MokŸev and fellow athlete and friend Kristina Khaleeva at an athletics meeting in Tula, a city 180 miles north of their home city, Kursk.

Yuliya's relationship with her coach was difficult and complex and it would end badly. Here MokŸev poses with a giant-sized champagne bottle at a homecoming celebration in Kursk after Yuliya's bronze medal performance at the European Indoor Championships in Paris, 2011.

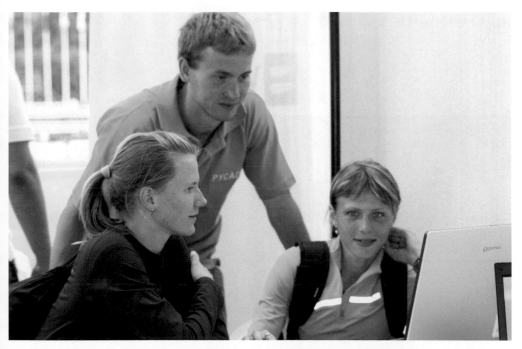

This was the July day in 2009 that Vitaly Stepanov first met Yuliya Rusanova. Yuliya's friend Oksana Khaleeva (left) was there to witness it.

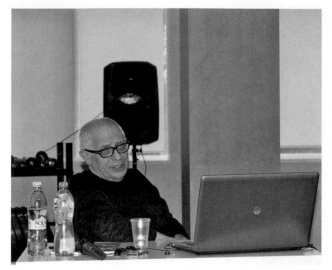

Doctor Sergei Portugalov was regarded as an expert on doping and anti-doping and a key figure in Russia's state-supported doping programme.

Grigory Rodchenkov (left), who would later become an important whistleblower, is seen here with Rusada's Vyacheslav Sinev during the time when both were part of the country's state-supported doping system.

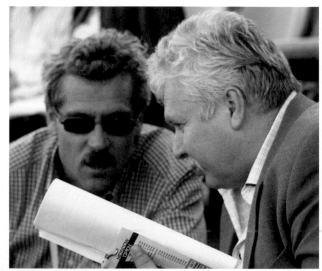

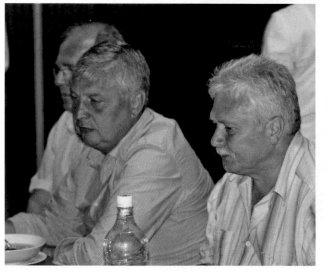

Former head coach in athletics Alexei Melnikov helped make Russia's doping programme work. Here's he with the then Rusada director general Sinev.

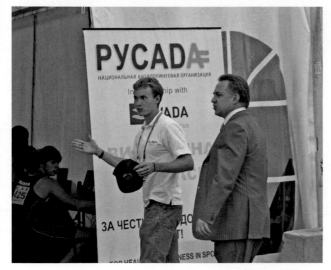

Together at the 2009 World Junior Canoe and Kayak Championships in Moscow, the then sports minister Vitaly Mutko and the then Rusada employee Vitaly Stepanov. They shared first names but not much else.

Rusada staffer Oleg Samsonov with Mutko in August 2009. Samsonov would later die in prison, Mutko would go on to become deputy prime minister.

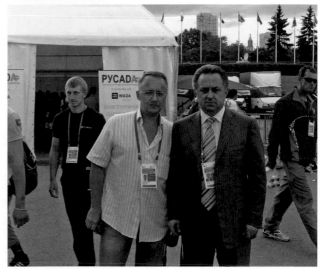

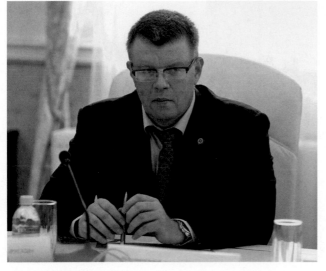

The former head of the Russian Anti-Doping Agency Nikita Kamaev died suddenly in February 2016. Fifty-two years old, Kamaev collapsed after returning from a morning cross-country ski. It was reported he had suffered a fatal heart attack. Many were suspicious of the circumstances surrounding his death.

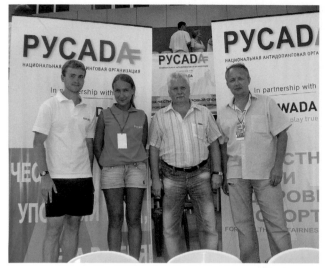

Rusada turned up in force at the 2009 Russia National Athletics Championships in Cheksobary. From left, Vitaly, Elena Ikonnikova, Vyacheslav Sinev and Oleg Samsonov.

At the 2009 World Junior Canoe and Kayak Championships in Moscow, Vitaly Stepanov and his colleagues flag up the collaboration between WADA and Rusada for health and fairness in sport. Behind the slogans, the reality was different.

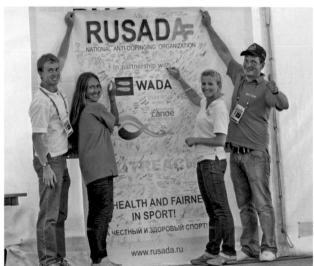

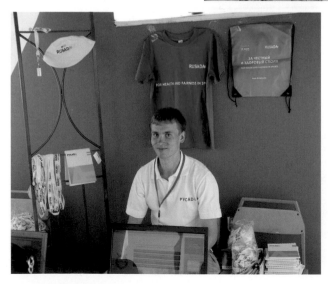

At the 2010 National Athletics Championships in Saransk, Vitaly mans Rusada's Outreach booth.

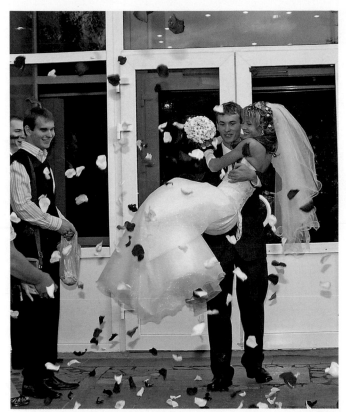

They'd known each other for barely two months but on 10 October 2009, Vitaly Stepanov and Yuliya Rusanova tied the knot in Kursk.

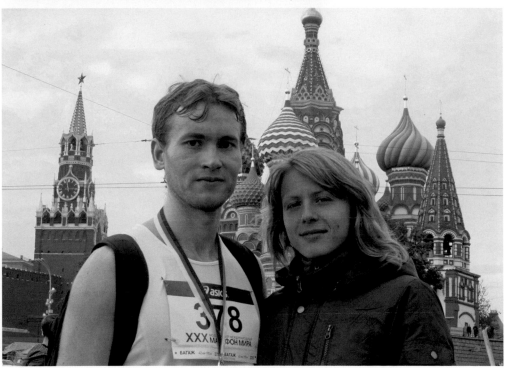

Vitaly has just run a marathon, Yuliya was there to support him. In the background, the building with the clock is the Kremlin. The other building is the impressive St Basil's Cathedral.

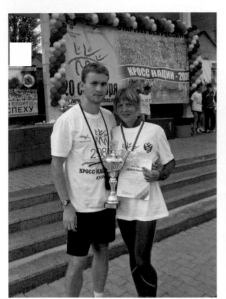
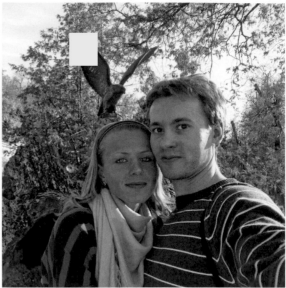

(Left) Yuliya has finished second in a road race at Kursk and has the trophy to prove it. Vitaly doesn't appear overly excited. (Right) Yuliya and Vitaly in front of a bronze eagle statue in Kislovodsk.

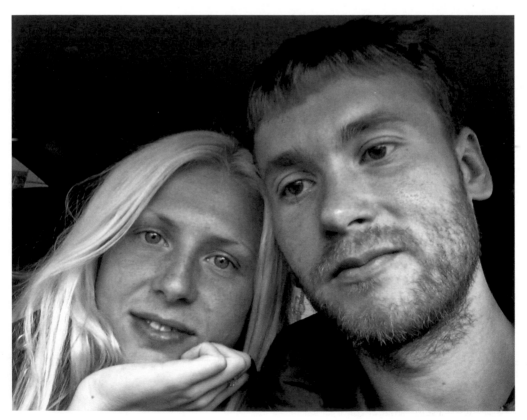

During the first three years of their marriage, there were moments of calm for Vitaly and Yuliya during the endless storms. This was September 2012.

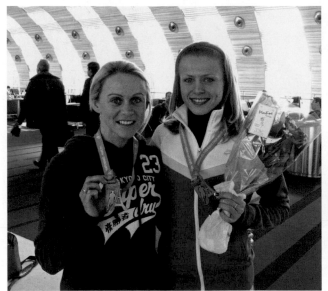
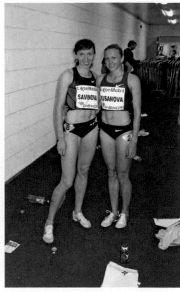

(Left) English athlete Jenny Meadows was one of the few non-Russian runners that Yuliya got to know. Here they are together at a Paris airport after the 2011 European Indoor Championships. (Right) Mariya Savinova and Yuliya at the Bislett Games in Oslo, June 2011.

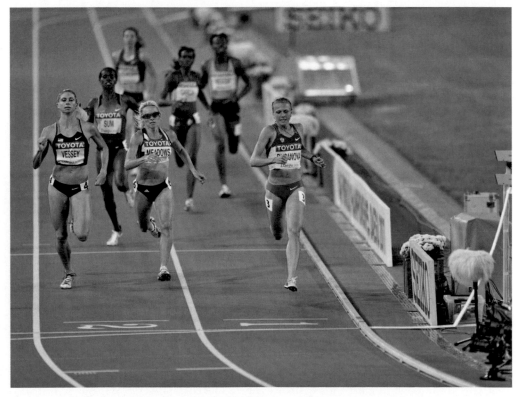

Yuliya wins a semi-final at the 2011 World Championships in Daegu. The American runner Maggie Vessey pipped Jenny Meadows in the race for second, thus costing the British athlete a place in the final, an outcome Yuliya was genuinely sorry about.

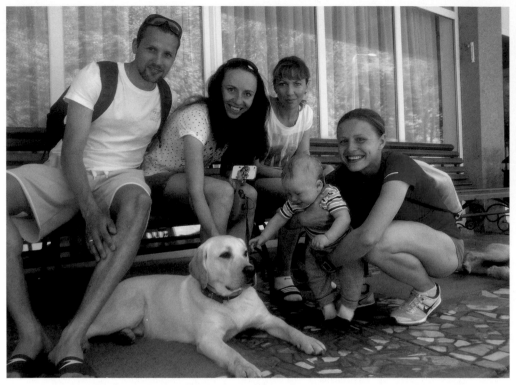

The difficulty for Yuliya (right, holding son Robert) in secretly recording those involved in doping came when she had to record her friend Mariya Savinova (second left), seen here with her husband Alexey Farnosov and fellow athlete Ekaterina Sharmina. The Savinovas' dog is Joy.

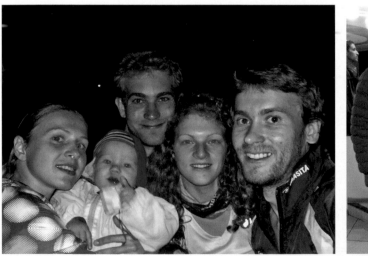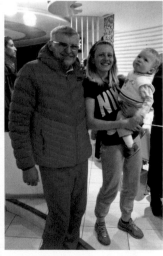

(Left) Yuliya, Robert, Vitaly's brother Igor and Igor's partner Olga Ermolova and Vitaly in Moscow. (Right) This will always be a special day for the Stepanovs, as it was Robert's first birthday, celebrated at a training camp in Kyrgyzstan. Robert's birthday party happened at a time when Yuliya was secretly taping her coach Vladimir Kazarin, pictured here, and her teammates.

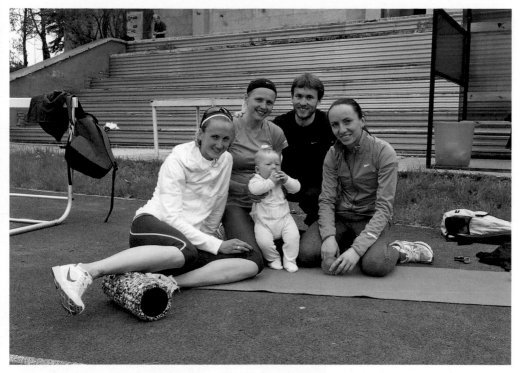

At a training camp in Kislovodsk in May 2014: Ekaterina Poistogova, Yuliya, Robert, Vitaly and Mariya Savinova. At this camp, Yuliya was gathering evidence that would later shock the world of sport.

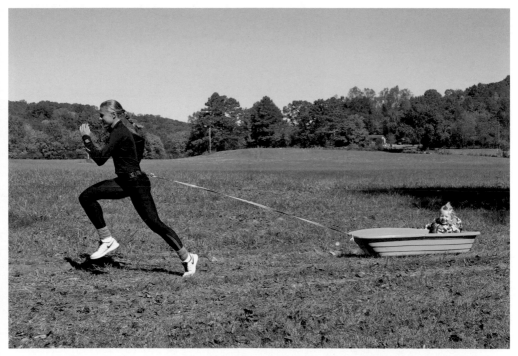

Robert, not yet two years old, provides some ballast for mum Yuliya's strength training.

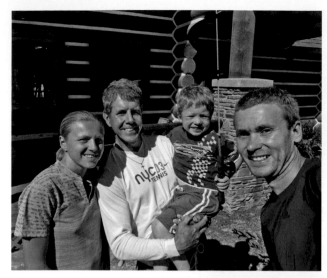

During his time as WADA's chief investigator, Jack Robertson brought Hajo Seppelt and the Stepanovs together and remained supportive of the whistleblowers after their story was broadcast. Here Robertson and the Stepanovs are together in the US.

Seppelt, the German investigative journalist, did a fine job in bringing the Stepanovs' story into the public domain and inspired the investigations that would lead to the banning of Russia from international sport. This is Vitaly and Hajo in 2015.

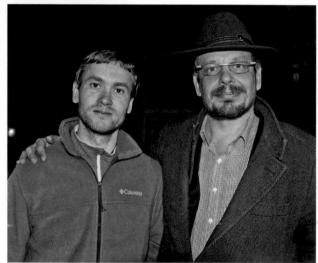

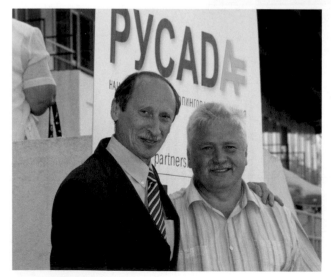

Valentin BalakŸichev (left) and Vyacheslav Sinev. On the day that German TV broadcast *Top Secret Doping – How Russia Makes Its Winners*, BalakŸichev was treasurer of the IAAF and president of the Russian Athletics Federation. He was soon forced to resign from both.

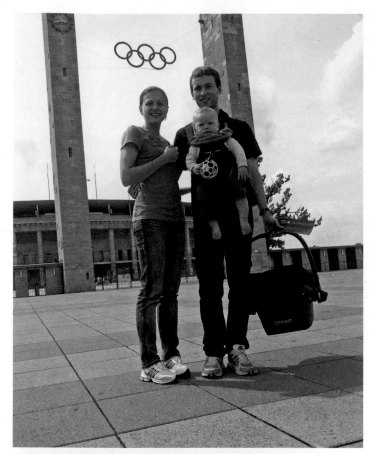

The Stepanov family standing in front of the Olympic Stadium in Berlin.

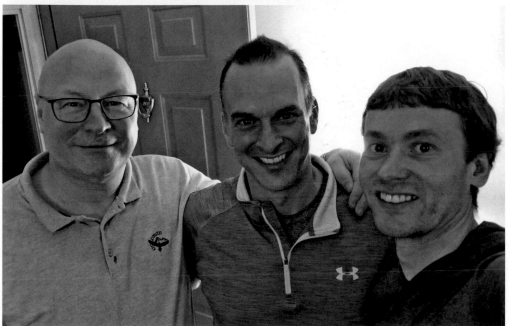

Patrick Magyar (left) and USADA chief executive Travis Tygart have been hugely supportive of the Stepanovs since they fled Russia in 2014. Here they are photographed with Vitaly.

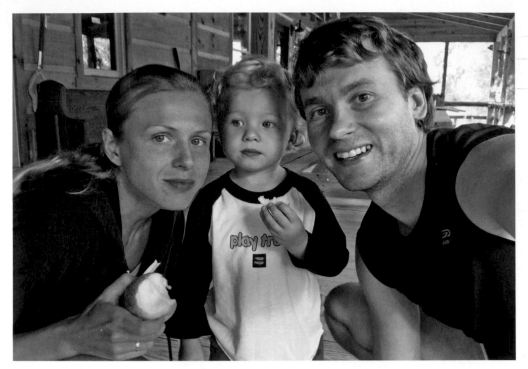

Yuliya, Robert and Vitaly are now in the US, awaiting the decision from US authorities that will determine their futures.

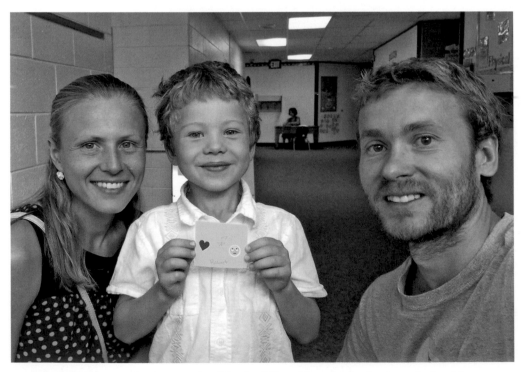

Robert started primary school in the US and here he is photographed at his school with Yuliya and Vitaly.

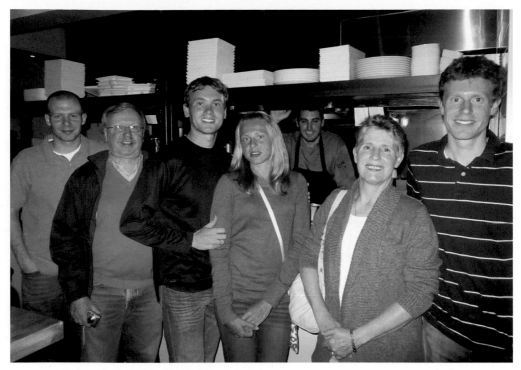

The Stepanovs surrounded by their American 'family' and friends. From left, Matt Hiestand, Jared Markowitz Snr, Vitaly and Yuliya, Andrew Parassio, Mary Helen Markowitz, Jared Markowitz.

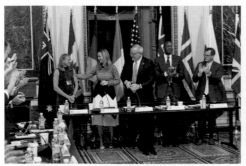

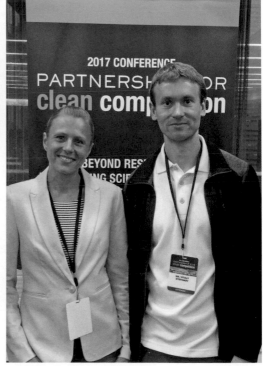

(Above) After Yuliya spoke to a White House committee in October 2018, she was astonished to be given a standing ovation by those present. (Right) In 2017, Vitaly and Yuliya were invited to a Partnership for Clean Competition conference in New York. Yuliya was presented with an award in recognition for her 'courageous and historic contribution to clean sport'.

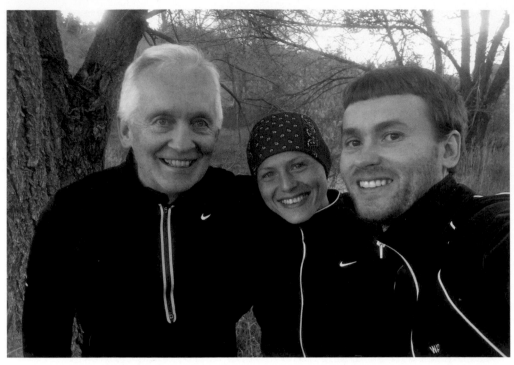

The author with Yuliya and Vitaly Stepanov on a winter's day in the US.

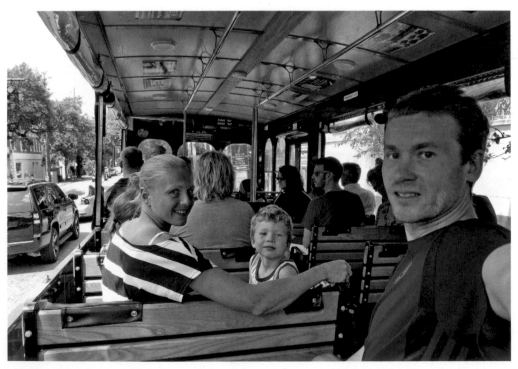

Before they set out on this city tour of Savannah, Vitaly didn't want to go.
Yuliya insisted, but before the end, Vitaly was glad he'd made the effort after making
a special discovery that summed up his journey.

He could choose to believe her. Or he could fuck off. He had chosen to believe but now there was no space left for belief.

They had some money saved. About $40,000. Maybe some more. Maybe as much as $50,000. Athletics money. Her money. It wasn't in the bank yet, it was just resting in the safe in the apartment. Vitaly decided he should have custody of the money. Her money. So while she slept, he checked his phone. As she had drunk her wine, he had recorded every word.

If you want to see your money again, Yuliya my sweet, you can fight me for it. Bitch.

The next day she had to go for therapy and rehab. She had tried doing hard workouts again and her thigh muscle was nagging. Because she asked him to, he drove her to the clinic. Then he drove straight home again. He removed all the money from the safe then drove across Moscow to the apartment of his relatives. He handed them a large brown envelope within a folder.

'Documents,' he said. 'They're mine. Can you keep them safe for me?'

He was back waiting outside the clinic again by the time Yuliya finished therapy. Later that day she left the apartment to go to stay with her mother, the formidable Lyubov, who was visiting relatives in Domodedovo. The next morning, Vitaly came home after a night in the taxi. Yuliya and Lyubov were in the apartment. The safe was open. Gaping and empty.

'We opened the safe and there is no money.'

'What money?' he said. 'You have the keys but you are asking me where the money is?'

She has been lying for three years, he told himself. *You can lie for one day, Vitaly.* Having the money would give him back some power. He'd have a last hold on her, a flimsy tenuous connection but for now it would do.

'You have the key, Yuliya. You have opened the safe. You

probably took the money and now you are blaming me because that's the way you are.'

'You,' said Yuliya's mother with blue murder in her eyes, 'are the worst person in the world.'

He stared back, stupefied. Where to begin with a response? Wasn't this the woman whose husband had murdered her father?

Later in January the oddest thing happened. Vitaly could hardly keep track of Yuliya's training camps at the best of times. Kazarin's group seemed to move from city to city like a band of gypsies. Now the group were training in Chelyabinsk of all places. Yuliya went shopping for food in an area called Rodnichok. In a city of one million people, in a part of town they rarely visited, she ran into Vitaly's parents.

She hadn't told them she was in Chelyabinsk. Vitaly hadn't told them either. For months Sergey and Elena had heard nothing from their son in Moscow. Yuliya and Vitaly were supposed to be shacked up in the big city. Sulky after the row over selling the family apartment but otherwise, as far as anybody knew, all was fine. Now here was Yuliya. In Chelyabinsk. What was she doing here? Why didn't she call?

'You must come to see us, Yuliya.'

Yuliya explained the gulag-like rigours of training camp. This shopping she was doing was a brief reprieve. Her life was just training and recovering. There was no time to be a social butterfly. She hoped they understood. She texted Vitaly later. Furious as if it were his fault.

'Your parents don't even know we are divorcing?'

And the Stepanovs called their son in Moscow. He saw their number come up on the phone. He had no answers for what they would ask. He could lie but why bother? He ignored their calls. He would find a good job and move out of their precious apartment. Then they could all do whatever the hell they liked.

Meanwhile, the whispers about the list of ninety-five athletes went on. Yuliya felt she would be among those banned. Melnikov was not sure. Perhaps she would be spared. Talks were ongoing.

'Maybe, Yuliya. Maybe not. It's a process.'

She was due to begin a course of anabolic steroids under Kazarin's supervision. She was looking forward to it. Since Kazarin had coached Mariya Savinova to win gold in London, everybody felt the same. 'I'll have some of whatever Mariya's having.' Then word came from Moscow instructing Kazarin not to proceed with the steroids until the sanctions issue was resolved. No point in pouring good drugs into somebody who is going to be banned.

Suddenly everything felt quite serious. The horse trading was nearly done. Yuliya had been sold.

Later, they learned how the trading was done. The Russian Athletics Federation had stepped aside. An IAAF representative sat down with Natalia Zhelanova, the woman in charge of the sports ministry department for anti-doping and interdepartmental co-operation. They went through the candidates, one by one.

This one's a no-hoper. Sanctioned.

This one's over the hill. Sanctioned.

Olympic champion? She's good. Mark her as clean.

European champion? Fly free, little bird.

'Yuliya Stepanova?'

'She is injured.'

'Okay. So, doper?'

'But on the other hand she is a prospect . . .'

'Clean, then?'

'But the husband. He is trouble, that one.'

'Let's come back to her . . .'

Vitaly had made a decision of his own. His war on doping wasn't over. He had nothing left except his convictions. Maybe

WADA could employ him? Or IDTM, the testing agency? He sent out CVs and covering letters. Despite the pending death of their marriage, he was still interested in Yuliya's case. He wrote again to Stuart Kemp. Kemp didn't answer. He couldn't comment on individual cases. But Vitaly kept asking. He couldn't help it.

~

Yuliya came back again to Moscow for one or two days and left again. He knew she was in town. She called him once or twice. He ignored those calls too.

January became February. Suppose he and Yuliya confirmed their divorce on 8 February? He had no job and the chances were that she would get a two-year ban. Was this not a time to be together? Was it not written in all the stars, in all the tea leaves, in all the cards of the fortune tellers? He was thirty years old and not getting any smarter. He still had to find a decent job, finally finish his education, just move on to the main chapter of his life, but he was unable to make any decisions. In the mornings he thought: *The fairest thing is to split the money. That is what we will do.* By the afternoons he thought: *She is not getting one damn rouble.* By bedtime he thought: *She made that money. I didn't make a cent of it. It is hers. All hers. What have I done?*

Yuliya was in some place down in Ukraine, a resort by the Black Sea, getting a mud treatment or some such. He called her. It was a short conversation.

'I am packing all of your belongings and driving them to Kursk.'

He pulled all the seats down and filled the car from bottom to top. Still he couldn't squeeze everything in. It took him ten trips up and down from his second-floor apartment to fill the car. There was so much stuff in the car that the rear-view mirror was redundant. Kursk was an eight-hour drive each way. He made the journey with lots of Coca-Cola and sunflower seeds to keep him going. Lots of overtaking to keep everybody else alert. Often he couldn't decide if it was the Coke or the fear of a head-on collision with a truck that kept him awake. Onwards!

He got to Kursk and called Yuliya's younger sister, Gelia.

'I am going to take this stuff of hers out of the car and put it by the entrance to your apartment building. What you do with it is your problem. Okay?'

Gelia still lived in the old family apartment on the fourth floor. It took Vitaly twenty minutes to unload the car. He left as soon as it was done, thinking that somebody had best move quickly to get Yuliya's stuff upstairs before it was scavenged. This place had some of the meanest streets he had ever seen.

Driving back to Moscow was hard. He didn't feel as good as he'd hoped to feel when he first planned the trip. Whatever closure was, he wasn't feeling it. Why was nobody shouting stop? Why were neither of them saying let's talk?

He got back to the apartment in Moscow. He called her. He'd been crying.

'We are family, Yuliya. You and I.'

'I really don't care, Vitaly.'

So two or three days later he made the trip to Kursk again. More of her stuff to be dumped. This time he brought a friend, Vladimir, along. It was easier with company. He told Vladimir about the money. Vladimir was hard-line.

'Don't give her one single rouble, Vitaly.'

They discussed it over and over until they hit Moscow traffic on their return. It took three hours of crawling to get to Vladimir's apartment.

It wasn't just Vladimir. Vitaly had run the story of his troubled marriage past seven or eight other friends. Each one had offered the same advice. He was better off without her, they'd said. Vitaly was persuaded. As for the money, Vladimir still hadn't softened by the time he got out of the car. He wasn't for sharing.

'Not one fucking kopek, my friend.'

Vitaly would keep it all and on 8 February he would be divorced. One more failure.

Yuliya had announced that she didn't want to come back to town for part two of the divorce proceedings. He could sign the final documents on his own. She had moved on. Good luck to her.

It took two more hours to drive to his own apartment after dropping Vladimir off. By the time he got home he had decided he was going to give her all the money back. What had happened had happened. He could never be free of her while he had her money in his pocket. In the apartment it was sparse and it was cold. There was no trace of her now and that killed him.

It was 3 February. The next day twenty-four centimetres of snow fell on Moscow.

Chapter 22

Towards the end of January Yuliya travelled to Crimea. Her left thigh ached and the pain prevented from her running. Saki, an old spa town near the Black Sea, was famous for the healing powers of its mud. A coach from Vologda knew a hotel owner there and he got her a room at half price. Yuliya booked in for two weeks. She was looking forward to this. Some therapeutic time on her own. Nothing to disturb the peace. Throughout the first week she took the five-minute walk from the hotel to the treatment centre. Off with her clothes, onto the floor to be covered from neck to toe in mud. Blankets were placed over the top.

Sometimes she would drop off to sleep. Other times she just lay there, forgetting the things she didn't want to remember. In the mud, under the blankets, she felt warm and safe. Thirty minutes and then washed clean by a shower. No amount of soap and water could get rid of the bromine smell of the mud. It wasn't pleasant but it wasn't a big deal. The tightness in her thigh disappeared. Then the pain. By the beginning of the second week she was back running. Free of injury, and free of Vitaly, her life was welcomingly simple again.

Alone, there were times when her heart ached. That was true. Occasionally she missed Vitaly's calls. She'd grown used to the reassurance of him needing her more than she needed him. Mostly, though, she was positive. The hotel was nice. The mud had worked. Her body felt ready again.

On 4 February 2013, three days before the end of her break, she was resting up in her hotel room. It was a Monday evening. The phone rang. *Ha*, she thought, *Vitaly*. She answered. Wrong. It was Vladimir Kazarin.

'Yuliya, do you remember we spoke about the biological passport problem?'

'Yes?'

'Well, listen. Something's come up. You'll need to come here, back to the region, to sign some papers about your employment.'

'Just to sign papers? Why?'

'It'll be fine. It's a bump in the road. Just come. Sign the papers. We'll talk then.'

'Bump?'

'They can't fire you—'

'Fire me? That doesn't sound like it'll be fine.'

'Let me finish. You've got to apply to them to release you from your contract. Don't worry. The ban is just two years. We will support you. Just come. Okay?'

The call was brief. Nothing more to be said. This wasn't a bump, this was a wall. Her life had changed in that one moment. Who she was, what she did, all her plans. Her entire existence had been a servant to one master. She prepared for the next season. Trained for the next race. Got ready for the next training session. She lived a life measured in 400 metre splits. Running was what she did and what she was. Now what?

Alone in Crimea, clarity came. They'd been distancing themselves because they knew a two-year ban was coming. Rather than tell her straight up, they drip-fed the new reality. She wasn't going to be in the team for the World Championships in Moscow. They'd been abandoning her without her even noticing. Bastards. She hated them now. How they had cared for her when she was useful and then discarded her when she wasn't. All her life, men had used her. Mokhnev, Melnikov, Portugalov,

Kazarin. Men were interested in her body or her talent. One or the other or both. Did any of them give a damn about her?

She would sign Kazarin's bloody papers. She would demand whatever the system could provide to banned athletes. She would continue to play the game, but now she saw them all for what they were. She would take care of herself, thanks. Fuck them all!

She thought about Vitaly, her soon-to-be-divorced husband. He didn't want anything from her. Or whatever he did want was stuff she wasn't good at dealing with. She'd pushed him away. She'd barely tolerated him. She had been with others. And where had it all got her? She was heading towards thirty. Her prime was passing. She was barely married to a man whose name she had not taken, whose love she'd neither accepted nor reciprocated, a man who continued to love her.

Yuliya, she thought, *it's you. You have made a mess of your life. You and your decisions.*

She thought about Katia. Her older sister had got married when Yuliya was a teenager. Yuliya was nineteen when Sasha, her nephew, had been born. What age was he now, seven? She envied her sister, mother to a lovely boy. What did Yuliya have? No career. No marriage. No kids. She'd always wanted kids. But not until she'd finished running. Now running was finished with her for two years. And she'd finished with her husband. Life wasn't simple. It was stark.

She lifted the phone again and dialled. No answer. She waited a few hours and called again. Still no answer. Ten times she called. Each time no answer. Shit. Not good. Not good at all.

She should have seen it coming. At the November training camp in Kyrgyzstan, Kazarin had mentioned 'some problems'. It wasn't a conversation Yuliya had wanted. Earlier in the year he'd asked if she could show him the results from her ABP tests. And at his birthday party in Sverdlovsk two months before, one of his sons had struck up a conversation and asked her who she was.

'Ah! Rusanova,' he'd said when she told him her name. 'My father told me about you. You are the athlete who has problems with your blood passport.'

'What kind of problems? I don't know about any problems.'

Really it was just that she didn't want to know. All the time she'd been running away from the problem. Now, with nowhere left for her to run, the pieces of the puzzle fell into place. For months Portugalov, Melnikov and Kazarin had been acting weird around her. Not as interested in her as they had been. She felt like she'd picked up some virus they were determined not to catch. At the time she had put it down to Vitaly. He was certainly something they didn't want to catch. Or didn't want catching them. They didn't like seeing him at training camps. Or maybe it was Mokhnev they didn't like. He talked too much. She knew that.

In this way, Yuliya had deluded herself.

~

Vitaly saw her number flash up a few times and he just didn't answer. He wondered about it, though. What was she playing at? He had just reconciled himself to the fact that he too would have to move on. And now she was calling him, screwing with his head?

On 5 February he went shopping with Vladimir. The winter was unusually harsh even for Russia. He bought himself a warmer overcoat against the brutal cold. It was more money than he'd ever spent on an item of clothing. They took in a movie together. Some mindless American thriller with bad dubbing. Vladimir was tugging him gently into the real world. Vitaly recognised his friend's intent. He wasn't pushing back. Anyway it was Yuliya's money that had paid for the coat and the cinema. She could pay for his retail therapy.

On 6 February she called again. On Skype. This time he
answered. She said she was in trouble.

'Are you?' he said. 'And now you're confusing me with somebody who gives a damn?'

'I need to talk to you, Vitaly.'

His head erupted like a broken truce; the peace he had established in his head was broken. Was she making fun of him? He
listened in wounded silence. The resentment was still frozen at
the bottom of his heart. He wasn't letting that go. Why was she
telling him? What about the boyfriend? The one who listens?
She kept on. She didn't know what to do. She said she was calling him because it was definite, she was about to be sanctioned.

'Yes? Well, let your lover-boy sort it out for you.'

She was scared, she said. She had fucked up. She was wrong.
She needed him.

He hated this. She'd had him at 'sanctioned'. She'd had him
when he decided to answer the call. She'd always had him. Any
fight he offered was just a fig leaf for his dignity. She talked
about the new boyfriend. Brutally honest, as always. Okay.
Sure. She had asked the guy about marriage. Or at least they had
discussed marriage. But her angle was clear. The new boyfriend
had been brutally honest too. He was not interested. He had
flicked her away like lint from his sleeve.

Ha, thought Vitaly. *Ha, ha, fucking ha!*

He had seen this guy or the version of this guy on his social
media. He was another 800 metres runner all right. From down
around the Chelyabinsk region too. Even by the high standards
of social media narcissism, he stood out as a self-involved idiot.
Anyway Vitaly didn't want to discuss him now. He didn't want
to think about him. He just wanted to tell Yuliya that he felt
her pain and he was really glad that it was her pain. She was
welcome to it.

'Vitaly,' she said, 'I don't know what I am doing with my life.'

'I know that. And again, it's not my problem. You left me.'

She kept coming back. She wore him down. She knew his vulnerabilities. His 'knight in shining armour' complex. In his heart he had wanted this chance. Let her fall on her face. Then let him scoop her up. He allowed her to unspool the details of the sanction. Coach Kazarin calling her by phone, asking when she was going to be in Moscow. Whenever she got to Moscow she needed to go and see Melnikov. Urgently.

She told Vitaly that maybe she had made a big mistake about divorce. Maybe neither of them should go to the registry office on the 8th. His mind was melting. They spoke for an hour and a half. Mainly he listened while she spoke.

There had always been something about the way in which Yuliya loved him – or, more specifically, the way she withheld her love from him – that had made him look forward to each day with her. When their relationship was trench warfare he kept walking forwards to be mowed down. Feeling anything was better than being numb. This strange woman would wave the white flag to him some day, he'd believed. In the end she would love him back. Now it was happening. Now she needed him if he could find the grace to accept her. *The grace? Wake up, Vitaly*, he thought. *Have you the desperation? The death wish? The foolhardiness? The complete lack of any dignity?* On the other hand, this call couldn't be that easy for her. Not after all this.

'Your mother,' he said out of the blue.

'What about my mother?'

'She was against our marriage.'

'So?'

'Well, here is what I want you to do. You talk to *my* mother. After you talk to her, if she tells me I am a fool then we will say goodbye. If she says to me, "Vitaly, you should take Yuliya back," I will take you back.'

'Call your mother?'

'Yes.'

'Okay.'

How odd, he thought to himself later. *I pick up the phone to tell her to go to hell and I end up asking her if she will have a conversation with my mother. Where did that come from?* It was not his first U-turn but it was the least explicable. He himself hadn't spoken to his mother in months.

Yuliya didn't have to ask Vitaly why he wanted her to ring Elena. She knew. All his adult life, all the way back to the failed America experiment and his squandering of their money, his parents had expected him to come unstuck. He starts a course, he leaves. He gets a job, he quits. He gets married, he's divorced. Yuliya knew he hadn't spoken to his mother for months. She knew he wanted his mother to know that this time it wasn't him. That they had come to the edge of separation because of Yuliya's actions, not his. He wanted her to be the one to explain this to his mother.

And maybe Vitaly had just wanted a checkpoint. A speed bump. *It's not that easy,* he was saying. But it was a punishment too: *talk to my mother because I know this is something you won't want to do.* Also: *you can't walk in and out of my life that easily.* And it was tit for tat too: *talk to my mother because your own mother cared about the money in the safe more than she did about anything else, but my mother will care about what is best for us.*

It was all those things, but mainly he was asking her how badly she wanted them to stay together. And by not needing to ask why he wanted her to call his mother, Yuliya had already passed part of the test. She had understood. Yuliya had never once called Elena during her marriage to Vitaly. They had yet to have a serious conversation. This wasn't the circumstance in which Yuliya would have chosen to break the ice, but it had to be done. The call lasted fifteen minutes. Elena was wary; her daughter-in-law was a mystery to her. Yuliya offered an account of a marriage that had known a lot of bad times and she told Elena that she, Yuliya, was the reason for those bad times.

'I have been a bad person.'

Elena listened with incredulity. She'd assumed that Vitaly would be the problem. Wasn't he always the architect of his own disasters? Yuliya said that she had been unfaithful. She had wanted a divorce so that she could begin again without any lies. Now she had a two-year ban and, honestly, she was scared. What was she to do? The decisions she had made, should she reverse them? Maybe she and Vitaly should stay together and start a family?

Elena wept at the other end of the phone. This was too much and too brutal. When she finally composed herself, Elena told Yuliya about how Sergey had been unfaithful to her. How she had forgiven him and they'd got through it. They'd stayed together. Elena's belief was that those God brought together belonged together. She told Yuliya she hoped that she and Vitaly would recommit to their marriage and carry on. The words were what Yuliya had been hoping for.

Vitaly didn't know exactly what had been going through Yuliya's mind since they spoke to each other but on 7 February she had spoken to his mother. That was something. But, having asked that it be done, he wondered now if it was enough. When somebody grabs the first offer you make, you always feel as if you should have inspected the goods a little more closely. Perhaps she was just keeping her options open and Vitaly was still in a neck-and-neck race with this Vladimir, the callow young 800 metres runner from Chelyabinsk. Vitaly weighed up his pros and his cons.

Pros. More mature. Use of family apartment. Some good times. Loyal. Already married to Yuliya. Not an alcoholic.

Cons. No job. No education. Not as good a runner as this Vladimir. Plenty of bad times. Unlikely to have his own apartment soon. Informing on Yuliya's doping practices to WADA. Unsure and confused about Yuliya's feelings. Unsure yet again about his own feelings.

As Vitaly saw it, he was off the lead but he was gaining. The other guy had no interest in marriage. It seemed now that marriage meant something to Yuliya. Not marriage specifically to Vitaly, but the idea of marriage generally.

On the morning of 8 February hc met her at Kursky railway station. It bothered him that he was always pleased to see her even when there was nothing in her eyes to suggest the feeling was mutual. He met her coolness with a blankness of his own, waiting to see how it would play out.

There was an exhausted post-war feel to their talk. As if life had drained the fight from her, and all the atrocities of their relationship had somehow become history. After their conversation, he sensed there were only two possible outcomes. They would either commit to making something of the marriage they had thrown themselves into, or they would never see each other again.

He drove her home, wondering if she ever even considered this place to be home.

Later they left the warm fug of the apartment to drive to Melnikov's office so that the sword might drop on Yuliya's career. Vitaly spoke as he drove. He said that he had been consulting Stuart Kemp via email. Kemp was cautious, as always, but Vitaly had been thinking. Yuliya's career was about to be destroyed because she was injured and expendable. Other athletes would be spared because of what they might bring home from major meets.

In this way he felt sorry for her, he said. He'd always been able to see Yuliya's life through her eyes. Running held that life together. They were so different in that respect. When it came to sport, Vitaly's talents amounted to a bit of everything and not enough of anything. He played for fun and friendship, and he ran because he knew that, without running, he was a lesser version of himself. Running was a good thing. In contrast, he continued, Yuliya wasn't just talented. Running gave her the things that ordinary civilian life couldn't give her. It gave her self-esteem. It made her somebody. It gave her a glimpse of a better place. For Yuliya, running wasn't a luxury. Running was the life-support system for her dreams. She felt like a real person when she ran. Real people had possibilities and choices.

Now the bastards who had given her running had betrayed her, he said. They had taken this one shining thing she was good at and told her she would be better at if she took the pills and suffered the injections. They had sensed her dread that she would be not be a runner without their drugs. That she would be nothing at all if she didn't take what they offered. They had rigged the game so well. And now she expected they would exploit that old dread in new ways.

Yuliya half-listened to Vitaly's summary as they drove through the snow. From today all racehorses would no longer be equal. Whatever she'd thought in the past, she knew that now he was right. She was being put out to pasture. She had used running to map her route to a better life. They were going to close that route down this morning. They were going to take running away from her this morning. Switch off the machine.

And then, in the afternoon, perhaps she would be divorced. They had spoken only of running and the drugs and the ban. It seemed to her that Vitaly required this business to be done before they moved on to the matter of divorce. He had said nothing about her conversation with his mother, about the grim appointment hanging over them later, about the future. By the evening she might have nothing except a return ticket to Kursk. This man beside her, he was still gabbling away. She had never needed him more. She had never loved him more. The thing was, he was the only man who truly cared for *her*. But now he was giving her nothing. No signs. No warmth.

From Vitaly's point of view, he was glad to find her not arguing back as he explained things. He had come to expect resistance. The truce of their married life had always been shakiest when doping was the topic. Now, though, she was agreeing with him by her silence. It seemed they shared a sense of outrage.

He continued to talk about WADA, casting the organisation as a protective relative. WADA knew what was happening, he told her. WADA knew this was wrong. WADA had its code, though. That code was incompatible with the Russian situation and the Russian code. Did she see? Was she getting this? Something different was needed, no?

She stared ahead into the grey light of the Moscow morning.

He spoke about the fight. He spoke about enough being enough. He spoke about his plans. He pulled in, and looked at her for affirmation or dismissal.

She nodded. Inscrutable. Forlorn. Small. Cold.

Still his wife somehow.

Chapter 23

'It's not me,' Yuliya had often told Vitaly. 'It's you.'

Now Melnikov sat behind his handsome desk in the Federation offices and looked at the woman whose career he was about to terminate.

'It's not us, Yuliya,' he said. 'It's you. And the rest of the world.'

Mainly, though, it seemed it was not them. He had a list. This list was a curse of a thing. It was being talked about all over Russia. It was his tragedy to have this list. Had she heard about some of the names on the list? This runner was banned. This one too. Tsk. Melnikov shook his head at the unfairness of it all.

'Anyway, now they're accusing us. They are saying that from 3 March 2011 . . . that was the Europeans, Paris, wasn't it?'

'Yes.'

'And up to March 2012, the results were unusual and are above the 99.9 per cent probability level, and that we have used a banned substance or method. They have sent a chart. With the results.'

Yuliya sat with her small bag on her lap. Fidgeting as Melnikov ran his finger over a graph, a doctor explaining the cause of death to a layperson. His words passed over her. They fluttered out the window. They hovered near the ceiling then floated like grey feathers to the floor. Nothing landed in her mind. It was done. She was moving on already and these were just words. *Haemoglobins and stimulation indexes and off-scores . . .*

very big discrepancy . . . didn't look good, of course . . . not even possible to go to a tribunal or a panel of experts with such varied results . . . 45.7 to 127 . . . crazy numbers.

How had they let this happen to her? She was off the scale at both ends. They were meant to protect her. Now more than ninety athletes had levels that made everybody look guilty and dumb. The Federation was hand-picking those who would be sacrificed.

Say what you have to say, she thought. *Stop making out this is just some act of God that has been visited on you.*

'I did everything you told me,' she said. 'And now . . . ?'

It was as if she had poked Melnikov with a stick. He didn't like her tone. Not after all he had done for her. He was still in his 'this hurts me more than it hurts you' mode.

'Okay, okay, hang on a minute,' he said defensively. 'Listen, this is what we'll do. The system we're talking about, we didn't really see the danger until spring 2012.'

'So now what?' she interrupted. 'How long do they want to ban me for?'

'The deal is this,' he said. 'Confess voluntarily, come out with your hands up, and probably two years. Just sign the document.'

Two years! If she contested, they said, she would get four years. That was why others had already signed. If she signed, her ban would be dated from the end of January 2013.

'I don't want it, Yuliya. Right to the very end, I did everything I could. I tried and that's it.'

Melnikov's tone was funereal now, sombre but reassuring at this difficult time. Out of respect, he would see to it that she got paid until the end of the year. She would be dead but still on the payroll. Until the end of the year at least. That would buy them time to think how they could support her. He would talk to Kazarin about continuing to train with them and run in relays.

As if that was a lovely and consoling thing. She saw his desperation for her to give him something. Some sign that she was grateful for what he had done and understanding of the failings that had brought everybody to this position. He wanted her to see that this passport system was a low shot. They'd told the coaches to stop but they wouldn't listen. The coaches thought wool was being pulled over their eyes all the time. He began to explain how, towards the end of the ban, she would be able to make a quiet comeback for Russia and be ready to shoot for the European Championships straight away. Suddenly he looked up.

'Kazarin!' he exclaimed, startling her as Vladimir Kazarin walked into the room.

What was her coach doing here? Melnikov seemed glad of the interruption. Yuliya had been depressing him. Now he boomed that Kazarin had been saying good things about Yuliya.

'Haven't you, Semenovich?' he said, using Kazarin's patronym to signify the warmth of the encounter.

As Kazarin gave nothing back, Melnikov trailed off. Mumbled something about rules.

'Tell me again,' said Yuliya. There was one thing she wanted clarity on. 'You are going to pay me just to the end of the year?'

'Yes.'

'And if I get pregnant? Will that make any difference?'

She would be doing them a favour, said Melnikov. Become pregnant by the end of the year and they would have to continue paying her. They couldn't eject a pregnant girl from the system. He was undertaker no longer. Now he was the oily host of a game show, happily announcing the bonus prize. But he had lost her attention again. Pregnancy? She had one man with no interest in marrying her. She had an actual valid husband outside in the car who was scheduled to divorce her after lunch. How had life got so complicated?

Melnikov was addressing himself mostly to Kazarin now but the words were for Yuliya's benefit. She had no idea what officials like Melnikov and Kazarin faced every day. Why, they would take a two-year suspension in a heartbeat. Sadly, that was not possible. They must go on. They counselled her to make the most of this time. When she came back they would pass on everything that had been learned.

'They're catching out people now who haven't even touched anything,' he said.

'It is ruined,' concurred Kazarin. 'Ruined.'

Melnikov asked Yuliya about her husband. The dope-testing guy. Was he working?

'Yes, he's working.'

'Where?'

'He found a job. He drives a cab.'

'So he's earning money?'

'Yes, it's okay.'

'So he's not going to say "I told you so"?'

'No, he won't.'

Melnikov found his rhythm now. Russia had been on its knees for ten or twelve years, he said. The factories had been shut down. Even the pharmaceutical ones had been running on empty. Now they were getting back, but developing any substance took time and billions. Not roubles but dollars. It was easier to find talent, like Yuliya or Savinova. They could do the job with the minimum of substances, so it made economic sense to develop athletes who worked off talent more than pharmaceuticals. Meanwhile the rules were changing. They weren't even looking for the direct presence of some substance any more, but they were watching how some protein behaved. And once that protein showed up, it was a case of 'let's have another look at you'. They called you back, all for this tiny, microscopic trifle. Ah, it was too much, too bloody much. What a mess.

'The document is on the table, Yuliya. Sign on for two years. You actually come out a winner.'

'I've got to sign now, right?'

'Yes, that's right.'

'And can I think about it?'

'If you want to, yes, think about it.'

'And can I take the documents?'

'Of course you can, they're yours.'

'And you'll be here on Monday?'

'Yes, I will,' she said.

'Just one thing: don't drag it out from all points of view. All in all, it'll allow you to come back in 2015 for the winter season.'

The document came sliding across the desk. They wished her all the luck and then watched her leave. Outside, in the car in the snow, she gave Vitaly the bones of it. Four years if she appealed and lost. The off-scores were so high she wouldn't win an appeal. And he'd said that if she got pregnant the time would really fly.

'Did you record it all?' Vitaly asked.

She removed her phone from her bag and nodded.

'Yes. Everything.'

Chapter 24

There was no divorce that day. They drove while discussing Melnikov and the problem of when she should she sign the papers that would formalise her ban.

'What do we do next now?' Yuliya said, softly stressing the *we*.

'Well, if you want to save the marriage we can try to save it. Or if you want to go to sign the papers we can go. So it is up to you.'

He spoke calmly, as if the question was one of takeaway food or just a sandwich at home. He didn't expect a quick answer.

What Melnikov had offered Yuliya was not unattractive. An American runner caught with a hand in the EPO jar would instantly lose sponsors and suffer social shame. But Yuliya was Russian, and in Russia something like this could happen to anybody. No big deal. There would be no stigma about the ban because Russians generally didn't care, and those who did care understood that doping was a requirement of the system. What athletes put into their bodies was low on the list of national anxieties.

Two years was a small amount of time and Melnikov had promised that he could compress it further for her. If there was a system to be observed there was a system to be gamed. And if she became pregnant Russia would guarantee that her income remained intact. If she preferred not to get pregnant, her income would survive in part anyway. Then there was Vitaly.

Melnikov hadn't said it, but nobody was going to miss having Vitaly haunting the training camps.

Right now, what was making everything worse was Vitaly's hardwired stoicism. She whipped him like a dog sometimes and he never bit back. He left no doubt that he loved her to the marrow of her bones. Nobody outside her family had ever treated Yuliya like that before and it tore at her soul. He didn't have to love her but he did. What was his game? If only he was some mean-spirited bastard like her dad. It would be so much easier to dismiss him. He talked about love and family while he survived on slivers of affection. She looked at his earnest face. Almost innocent. She'd tried to straighten him out with a haymaker of reality but he was still standing.

I am sorry, she thought.

Melnikov had understood the possibilities. Yuliya could walk away. But if she wanted her career, the system would wait for her the way a convict's wife waits for the convict. This was the system that had brought her into its circle of trust. Yet, for the next two years, it could do nothing much. She should keep in mind, though, that ninety-four other Russian athletes had been 'failed' too. It was nothing personal and she was nothing special. It was a foreign conspiracy and when it came to offering sacrifices to WADA, Yuliya unfortunately was a perfect fit. Promising but persistently injured and with a couple of last-place finishes in big races. She was young enough to bounce back from a two-year ban. It was tough for now. He knew that.

She had realised, listening to them talk, that she was suddenly sick of it all. The Melnikovs. The Portugalovs. The Mokhnevs. They were a syndicate of old men and she was their show horse. One filly in a vast stable. Life with them was all substances and no substance. Quality of life was for Americans.

'What about me?' she wondered. 'What about my life?'

Last week she had been hoping to marry a man she played

cards with at training camp. That's just about how happy and well adjusted she was. She'd wanted him to love her. She'd needed him to. He'd fled when he understood her neediness.

Vitaly loved her. Men wanted you to be playthings or punch-bags. You figured out which they wanted and you got on with it, taking happiness where you could get it. You survived men. Was that why it was so odd to be with a man who made it so easy? She tested him and taunted him and threw the truth at him like battery acid, but there was no flinch in him. Now he was asking her what would she like to do.

'Two years from now, five years from now, where do you want to be, Yuliya?'

Nobody ever asked what she wanted. Not really. What else did he have to prove to her? Was a man like this ever going to come into her life again?

'If you want to save our marriage,' he said, 'we can try to save it.'

She had no rights here. She'd come back broken and helpless. It wasn't him, after all. It was her all along. But he was taking no revenge. Forgiveness really was the scent the violet leaves on the heel that crushes it.

'Yes,' she said now, 'let's try to save this.'

Her life jackknifed again. It was 8 February 2013. She felt thoroughly clean.

PART THREE

'But what can be done, the one who
loves must share the fate of the one who
is loved.'

Mikhail Bulgakov,
The Master and Margarita

Chapter 25

Vitaly was excited. This was a side of him Yuliya had forgotten. She found it appealing. More so than his melancholy default mode. She liked this guy suddenly so brimming with intent. He transferred her tape of Melnikov onto his laptop and listened to just a little of the content. The sound quality pleased him and he knew instantly that the material was going to interest a lot of people.

This February day felt like another beginning for Vitaly. This tape and Yuliya's nerveless making of it was her present to him. It was as if events were honouring a long-standing appointment with the life he'd hoped for. Spring was budding early.

'Can I get in touch with Stuart Kemp tonight?' he said excitedly. 'You know, the guy from WADA? . . . Maybe we can go public . . . Probably if we go public it is better that we are not in Russia when it happens . . . We have our American visas so we could go there . . . Maybe in the next few days we should go to Kursk and bring back some of your things.'

She listened but didn't take it in. The day was throwing her in such random directions it was like tumbling in a washing machine. This evening she was no longer an athlete. She was staying married to the man she had been scheduled to divorce an hour ago. He was talking about going to America. It was not going to be a quiet life. Fine. She would meet it head on with her customary determination.

For the next four weeks the excitement never eased. She went with it all, clear-eyed and motivated. One day it seemed that she would complete her ban and return as a clean athlete, and the dealings she and Vitaly might have with WADA would remain anonymous. The next day they were on the verge of going public in a fireworks show of publicity, after which they would vanish and live happily ever after.

Vitaly spoke to Kemp again. Four days later they taped Melnikov again at the National Indoors. Why had Vitaly never thought of this before? Hanging them with their own words. Hoisting them with their own petards. Why had WADA never suggested it? It was simple and brilliant. The seed had been planted when he'd seen the panic in that joker Markovchin's eyes back in Kursk when he'd merely thought that Vitaly had taped his words. He'd coughed up Yuliya's money instantly.

Why wasn't WADA now more excited by this turn? Trying immaculate conception to produce the baby that Melnikov had suggested would be easier than coaxing an encouraging word from WADA. If life with Yuliya had been frustrating, dealing with WADA was a torture of unresponsiveness. Vitaly had often felt like sending them a short email. *Hello? Anybody there?*

After a murmur of initial excitement when Vitaly told them of the recordings, any official enthusiasm had subsided. They were still tied by their own code, they shrugged. What could they do? And, of course, they were hampered by concern for Vitaly and Yuliya. WADA's responses had reverted from mildly interested back to extremely cautious. This was all fine, they said, but a third party would have to be informed. There was now vague talk about arranging some sort of meeting so that Yuliya might tell everything to WADA, but they felt that the IAAF should be part of that meeting. To Vitaly's surprise, they actually seemed to see no problem with that even though, as any

Russian knew, the addition of more bureaucracy to any process just constipated that process.

For three weeks they had spent their evenings in the apartment, working on a long letter to WADA that would serve as an introduction to their new modus operandi. The letter was also a confession. Yuliya told the story of her life in running, tablet by tablet, injection by injection, test by test.

The writing gave her a new perspective. She put the words on the screen and Vitaly parsed them for her. For the first time she saw her life from outside herself. She'd thought she'd had choices when she'd merely been hurried along by her circumstance, desperate to get away from Kursk. She'd always been reacting to what was behind, always chasing what was ahead. The system hadn't found her. She had found the system. She'd gone looking. She'd wanted whatever they had to offer. She'd wanted to do whatever had to be done. There had been no deal with the devil at a crossroads. She'd been in too much of a headlong hurry to notice any crossroads. That was how they operated. They took your awful hunger and treated it with injections and pills.

It was unfair that she should be the one biting down on a cyanide pill now while Melnikov and Portugalov looked on with their crocodile tears and pursed lips, but commiserating with herself was to miss the point. It wasn't complicated. The system had to survive. If you chopped its head off, another head grew back in its place. If Melnikov or Kazarin put their hands up and offered to share any punishment, there would be a new Melnikov and Kazarin by Monday morning. Just like there would be a new blue-eyed young Yuliya prepared to do whatever it took.

Old Valery Kulichenko had bit down hard on his cyanide after the Tatyana Lysenko scandal back in 2007. He'd wailed like a big baby. He'd thought he was an essential cog in the machine, but he'd been removed and discarded while the machine never missed a stroke. Russian sport was the drinker who was forever swearing that he had cleaned up his act when in fact all he'd done was find a new hiding place for the vodka bottles.

Her letter to WADA concluded on a note of resigned realism. She transferred her trust to the Dudley Do-Rights with their conferences and their achingly rheumatic system.

'I understand that maybe the most that I can do is to share my story with you and continue living in Russian reality. It's like, I live in Russia by Russian rules and the doping fighting is in Canada. And Canada seems like a different planet at this point.

'If I cannot really change anything then I will try to fully recover from all of my injuries and become a mother. And in two years I plan to come back and do what I enjoy doing the most – run. I hope that in two years WADA will find a way to make a change in a better direction and I will be able to compete in Russia and internationally fairly.'

Two years? The anger stage had passed. She had moved on to acceptance.

~

While the first excitement of the recordings wore off, Vitaly and Yuliya took stock. They had a three-year history of mostly unhappy marriage. They had a future of some sort. Perhaps with a baby in it. They had a life in Chelyabinsk maybe. Vitaly had a notion to fix up some building there and to run a mini-hotel. (In a city that had always repelled visitors? Well, everybody loves a dreamer.) They had the prospect of a low-key life, quietly filling in the yawning gaps in WADA's childlike understanding of Russia.

Yuliya would not be an athlete for two years but she could

go to training camps and run for the police, who would give her a pension when her legs were marbled with varicose veins and her name was forgotten. The police were oddly indifferent about biological passports and failed dope tests. They had the police contract, money until the end of the year, and they had two tape recordings with incriminating words on them. The next step seemed obvious. They could make a baby or they could get more recordings and better recordings. Either activity would be something to keep them occupied.

Vitaly spoke to Kemp again. And again Kemp said to come and tell them everything he knew and that they would get somebody from the IAAF along. Habib Cissé was dealing with Russian cases.[1]

This was so disappointing. Again with the IAAF? Did the situation really need the very 'complicated' moral positions of the IAAF added to it?[2] Vitaly suggested that, rather than fly to the States to see them, it would be better to wait. In time, he and Yuliya would share everything they knew. In the meantime, their goal would be to gather more evidence. It had been easy to tape Melnikov and Kazarin. They would engineer opportunities to record bigger fish like Rodchenkov and Portugalov. Kemp had a second suggestion. One that didn't involve the IAAF, which was promising.

'Maybe you would like to talk with Jack Robertson.'

'Ah. Yes, that would be good. Where?'

'Istanbul?'

'Istanbul? Okay. Of course.'

They met Robertson early one morning in the lobby of the Renaissance Polat, close to Istanbul airport. This was a work trip made by three impatient people. There was no boating on the Bosporus, no bowed heads in the Blue Mosque or wasted nights in the Golden Horn. They came. They spoke with Robertson. They went home.

It had been a year since Yuliya had flown to Istanbul with the Russian team for the World Indoor Championships, their systems flushed pristine-clean under Portugalov's guidance. Two years had passed since Vitaly had sat in a Boston hotel with Robertson and others. Nothing had happened since. Another false start with WADA. Dealing with them was like that Samuel Beckett play where nothing happens, again and again.

Still, Vitaly viewed Robertson as the last chance of progress and was pleased to see him. They talked a lot. With near-forensic care they combed through the document Yuliya and Vitaly had spent three weeks writing, honing and translating. Robertson went over Yuliya's entire story as it had been documented. He had an investigator's mindset and had seen many things. Nevertheless, it was a surprise to read that one woman's small, compact body could have hosted so many pharmaceuticals and survived.

There were documents from doping control officers. Precise records of what Yuliya had taken. It was the true life of one Russian athlete in the stranglehold of the system. And the tapes. The tapes were a smoking gun.

Before there could be any solutions, though, there was an immediate problem. Yuliya and Vitaly had some bullets with them. At the end of 2012 Kazarin had spoken to Yuliya in Kyrgyzstan about her preparations for the forthcoming winter. He had given her steroids but then a minute later mentioned that she might imminently be sanctioned. Yuliya never took the course of steroids. Now they had brought the pills to Istanbul and handed them over to Robertson. Neither of them had seen *Midnight Express*. Robertson had to travel on to Canada as the next leg of his trip. He was now involved in an ongoing investigation. He was representing WADA. If he were to be stopped coming through Montreal airport carrying the Kazarin steroids from Turkey, he couldn't shrug his shoulders and say that somebody who would have to remain nameless had just given him the steroids at a meeting in Turkey. They'd brought them from Russia for him to take a look at and now he was taking them into Canada to do just that. Just a look, honest. We're the good guys.

Vitaly recalled travelling to Donetsk in Ukraine to perform a doping control at a professional boxing event. There was officially a border to be crossed when Vitaly was returning to Moscow on the train. Police would board the train and search the luggage of anybody they felt looked suspicious. Rusada hadn't, of course, supplied the documents to clear the way for doping controls to be transferred from Ukraine to Russia. So he had talked to Sinev and been told, 'Well, Vitaly, just hide the samples.' He had wrapped up his six samples in his clothing and stuck them at the bottom of the bag covered with more clothing. He made it through. Now here he was, handing over steroids that he had brought to Istanbul to pass to a former drug control enforcement officer now working for WADA.

Robertson was too consummate an agent to reveal his plan, but Vitaly suspected that he had one. And indeed he had. That evening in Istanbul, Robertson was meeting an old friend from the DEA days. When your Russian steroids absolutely, positively have to get there overnight, use the DEA Express.[3]

Robertson had entered the game and Vitaly left Istanbul hoping that everything would move a little faster from here on.

Chapter 26

Since the day of their near-divorce they had found a little glas-nost in their relationship. They talked as they had never really done about the future, each assuming that the other would feature in that future. They even talked about the idea of having a child as much as they talked about WADA. Having a child and giving it the love and all the other things Yuliya had never had. This had once been a dream of hers and, now that she took it down from the shelf, she recalled its warmth.

She and Vitaly. Big decisions and long hours talking about them. She felt safe.

Now, though, what to do? Where to live? How to live? Who to live with? With rent-paying flatmates or even with a hungry baby? Moscow was impossible. Vitaly's brother and his girlfriend had returned from their trip to Australia. Too much cabin fever came with being cooped up with them again. Kursk offered nothing. No work there and nobody who appreciated Vitaly's qualities.

There was always Chelyabinsk. In the good times Vitaly's parents had built a big house there as a project for their retire-ment. They had begun work around the turn of the century, hoping to create a mini-hotel, but their money had run out. Vitaly felt he was the person to take up the challenge of its restoration. The Hotel Stepanov? Why not? Moving to Chelyabinsk was a cheap option. They could work together there. In the second coming of their marriage, they found the romance of that appealing.

Regardless of Melnikov's pregnancy and income sermon, the idea of making a baby was attractive to both of them. So far they had lived parallel and often separate lives. A baby would sweep away the self-absorption that marked their warfare. A child could be the defining event of their relationship.

Money didn't need to be a factor. They had the money that Vitaly had stolen from the Moscow safe and had sheepishly returned a week or so later. He had simply returned the cash to the safe. No explanation was sought, and none was offered. As Melnikov had pointed out, Yuliya would be paid for the remainder of the year, and they had the income from the police. A baby would arrive because a baby would be wanted. It was decided. Yuliya, always quick, became pregnant almost instantly. As soon as the result of the pregnancy test was confirmed, she applied to have her name changed. That too happened quickly. Yuliya Rusanova became Yuliya Stepanova. So this was what commitment felt like? Who knew?

Apart from the large building with mini-hotel potential, Vitaly's parents also owned a nearby apartment in Chelyabinsk. It was in a sickly state of repair but it had possibilities. So, first Vitaly and Yuliya set about making a nest of that old apartment, a perfectly homely place to bring their baby home to. The Hotel Stepanov could wait.

One day in the car they were listening to a call-in radio show. They hushed each other suddenly and turned up the volume. The discussion was about a trend among Russians to go abroad to have their child. Specifically, people spoke about Russians going to Australia. Vitaly and Yuliya laughed. People! What a crazy idea. Australia! Mad.

A few months later Robert Stepanov was born in the USA. After ten heaving hours of labour at Reading Birth Centre, 30 miles west of Macungie, Pennsylvania, Yuliya was moved to Reading Hospital. There, Robert arrived via Caesarean section in a spotless, sunlit room with a retinue of smiling nurses and encouraging midwives attending.

This was just as Yuliya had imagined it when she had begun to dread another encounter with the haphazard Russian health system. Russian maternity centres, or *roddoms*, had mixed reputations. If you had money at all and you wanted adequate treatment, you were advised to bribe an obstetrician. The further you got from Moscow, the harder it was to find obstetricians worth bribing. In Russia pregnancy was still a problem to be treated, trouble brought to the door of the system. The more Yuliya had thought about the radio call-in, the more she had liked the idea. But not Australia. America. They knew people there. A child being born as an American had options. And she still had most of the money she had won or earned in her running career.

At the same time Vitaly was experiencing a little déjà vu. He had come back home to Chelyabinsk once before and it had been a mistake. Only a fool makes the same mistake twice. Now he'd concluded that they would never really have a mini-hotel there. It was his parents' house and it always would be, even if they let paying strangers in.

The conversation between Vitaly and Yuliya about America had been short. We are doing it! We are not telling anybody; we are just doing it! Nobody has to know. But we are doing this.

In America they found themselves at the door of a familiar inn. The home of Mary Helen Markowitz and Jared Markowitz Snr in Macungie, close to Allentown, Pennsylvania. The Markowitzes' hearts seemed as big as America itself. Much time had passed since Vitaly had come to stay with them in the months after 9/11. Their own children had all flown the nest. Now Mary Helen and Jared Snr shared the house with their beloved dogs, Wolfy and Chaucer. They lived quiet lives that they were happy to share. They opened their arms to the young Russian couple as if they were long-lost family.

They had been with the Markowitz family for two months when Robert came into the world. In that time, they ate well, slept well and got ready. It was perfect. Vitaly's old friend Jared would join them in his parents' house at weekends. Yuliya's English improved. They rented an old Kia Optima for $19.99-a-day from Rent-A-Wreck. They were happy.

As usual with Yuliya and Vitaly, nothing was simple. Vitaly was punctilious, as always. He wanted everything to be right. Entering America, he had made sure to tell the Customs and Border Protection official at the airport that his wife was pregnant, and then furnished documentary proof that he had the financial means to pay for the birth. He'd exhaustively researched all the options and he hoped Yuliya would be able to have the baby at a birth centre. If it was all plain sailing, that would cost $4,000.

The sailing was anything but plain. Paying for the move from birth centre to hospital was going to consume a large number of the crumpled old notes Vitaly and Yuliya had once fought over back in Moscow. They were looking at $4,000 for the birth centre then almost $10,000 for the hospital, excluding another $1,600 in anaesthesia costs. In these situations, Vitaly excelled.

The day after Robert was delivered with all those smiling nurses and doctors in attendance, Vitaly went to the hospital with some ibuprofen bought from a nearby Walmart. Once they were alone with their newborn son, Vitaly slipped the painkillers to Yuliya.

'Take these instead of what they try to give you. These cost ten cents. Theirs cost $7 for exactly the same pill.'

'Okay.'

'How are you feeling?'

'Sore but fine.'

'Would you be able to go back to the Markowitzes with Robert this afternoon?'

'Yes, I think so.'

When the doctor came round Vitaly spoke to him.

'Yuliya would like to go home this afternoon.'

'Twenty-four hours after a C-section?'

'Yes.'

'This is the first time in my experience that anyone has left hospital so soon after a C-section. Normally we recommend four nights for mothers who've had a C-section.'

'It's going to cost us another $2,000 if Yuliya stays one more night, and that's before she is examined by doctors, has her temperature taken by nurses, and receives whatever medication she needs. We don't have that kind of money.'

'Okay,' said the doctor. 'If your son's blood work is good, it is safe for your wife and son to be discharged.'

Back in Macungie, Vitaly set to work. He haggled like a Russian at the market. He made phone calls, wrote emails, and then followed up with more emails. He started with the birth centre. If a woman agrees to pay $4,000 for a birth to occur in the birth centre and then the birth doesn't occur in the birth centre, can that birth centre still demand $4,000 for the birth? They gave him $900 off just for the temerity of the philosophical enquiry. Elsewhere he promised the carrot of instant cash for discounts while wielding the stick of arguing over every single item on the invoices. He wore them down. In the end he saved $5,000.

The warmth of the Markowitz house got into their bones. Vitaly realised that this woman whom he had fallen so hard for was all that he had hoped she might be. She had hurt him, but he saw that as the toll he paid on the route to where he wanted to go. On that awful night back in the Moscow apartment when she had told him everything, all the bad and the ugly, he had made recordings of her speaking to him. He had never known why, or what he intended to do with them apart from wallow in their harshness, but they didn't exist any more now. He had destroyed them. Gone, too, were the thoughts that had once bothered him. He would forgive her anything and everything. And she would remain forgiven.

She began to see the good in this man. It surprised her that when she imagined him as some other woman's husband, she felt pangs of jealousy. Somebody else having everything that Vitaly stood for? That cut her. A good man was hard to find. She had made mistakes, but ultimately she had been blessed. She believed this was how it was meant to be.

And there was Robert, whose warmth welded them together. Yuliya initially liked the named Artem, meaning 'unharmed and in perfect health', but Vitaly had campaigned for something that didn't hint at any nationality. Robert was the fourth name that popped up on an internet name-generating game, and they knew instantly that was it. Robert.

When they talked about their future now, it revolved around Robert. Their plan was to bring their son back to Russia as soon as was possible. First, they had to get US and Russian passports for their son. The Russian general consulate in New York told applicants to expect a six-month delay. Problem. Vitaly and Yuliya's visas meant they had to leave the US before 13 March 2014. So Vitaly went to the grey building on 91st Street on Christmas Day. With 25 December not being a holiday in Russia, the consulate was open and Vitaly knew there would be no queues. He pleaded with a passport official for a speedier delivery. He explained that his wife's father was gravely ill and she needed to return home as soon as she could. It was true that Igor was unwell. True and convenient in this instance. Through the most difficult stage of the illness that would end his life, Igor

Rusanov was unwittingly helping his middle daughter. The application was placed near the top of the pile.

On their walks around Macungie with their new baby, they talked about Vitaly's almost three-year trail of emails to WADA, a trail that appeared to have reached a natural end with Robert's arrival.

'Yeah, I know it now. It was a waste of time.'

'I told you that the first time we talked about it. "Don't be an idiot," I said. Remember? There is a system and one small guy isn't going to change it. Even if he is Vitaly Stepanov.'

'It's just life. Just how it is. You live and learn.'

'We've got Robert to worry about now. So let them get on with it.'

They had brought Robert home to the Markovitz house in November. On New Year's Eve they were watching the TV coverage from Times Square. Giddy, beery revellers cramming the famous space and clogging the arterial streets, waiting for the familiar ritual. Countdown, crystal-ball drop, 'Auld Lang Syne' and then some Sinatra, *Start spreading the news . . .*

Six or seven minutes before midnight, Katia called from Kursk, where it was already 8 a.m. on New Year's Day. Yuliya went upstairs to take the call.

'Yuliya. It's Katia.'

'Yes?'

'Could you hand the phone to Vitaly?'

That was enough. She knew.

'It's our father?'

'Yes. He's died.'

She cried. Afterwards she wondered about that. It was her postnatal hormones, she told herself. They were all over the place. But it wasn't just that. Igor was still her father. There were good memories too. When the tears stopped she went downstairs and Mary Helen hugged her.

The details came the next day. Igor been staying with Grandma Alla. Yuliya's sister Gelia had been at his bedside. Around 2 a.m. Lyubov came so that Gelia could go out and enjoy the New Year festivities. An hour later, Igor complained to Lyubov about feeling too hot. He asked for the window to be opened. Still he felt too hot and unable to breathe. She opened more windows. He asked her to open the door. Then, before she could stop him, he got out of bed and began crawling towards the door. At the door, he collapsed. By the time Lyubov got to him, he was dead.

They flew back to Moscow late on the night of 13 February. People are strange in their superstitions. You can fly cheaper on the 13th. So they had left for America on Friday 13 September 2013 and returned on Thursday 13 February 2014.

The city was cold. Snow and sleet and business as usual. The Winter Olympics were on. They watched the Sochi Games with jaundiced eyes. Bright lights, big stars, gleaming buildings. Mother Russia in her glad rags, showing off for all the world to see. And Mother Russia topping the medal table too.

Vitaly shrugged his shoulders. It was all a big show but no one cared. Not WADA. Not the IOC. Not the sponsors or the TV companies or the journalists. He wasn't regretting his decision to leave all this behind him. Since the meeting with Jack Robertson in Istanbul, Russia had hosted the IAAF World Championships in Moscow and its doped athletes had won more golds than any other country. The first time a host nation had topped the medal table. Everyone had clapped on cue.

Three months later WADA held a conspicuous world conference on doping in South Africa, with 2,000 delegates there to talk shop and snaffle canapés. The organisation could easily have rebranded as Conferences 'R' Us. Hoping to pierce their leathery conscience, Vitaly had written another email to WADA during the conference. He received no reply. WADA was too busy conferencing about doping to worry about doping.

Around the same time Robert had been born and Vitaly had begun to suspect there were things in life more important than anti-doping. Yuliya had understood from the beginning. 'Don't be an idiot, Vitaly,' she would advise. She had switched sides, though. He was proud of that. And they were still a family. Not bad for an idiot.

Yuliya warmed to normal life. The clubs she was attached to continued to pay her. She didn't have to dope, and competing at elite level ceased to be an obsession. If she had a second child it would mean that under Russian law her income would be guaranteed for three years. The amount would be reduced but it would be enough. Somebody had told her once that in her future was a courtly fellow with whom she would have two children. This level of fiscal detail hadn't been included, though. She got on with the quotidian chores of Russian life. She registered Robert with the medical services to make sure he had his check-ups. She shopped. Cleaned. With Vitaly she passed time in Moscow traffic jams. They remained busy in the world and kind with each other. They had no complaints. There was a baby and optimism in their lives.

Apart from Vitaly's immediate family, nobody in Russia even knew that they had been out of the country. Yuliya had told her family and her coaches that Robert would be delivered in Chelyabinsk. When she came home to Russia, the fiction about his birthplace continued. Living in the largest country on the planet allowed you to pretend that you were always in some other room. It would be an easier start to Robert's life if he wasn't announced as the child who had been born in America so that he might have the privilege of dual citizenship. Anti-Americanism wasn't hard to find in Russia, especially in the world of athletics. To spare themselves any trouble, Robert was presented as a son of Chelyabinsk.

One evening in Macungie, Vitaly had sat up late, talking with

Mary Helen. He had told her at length about his dealing and frustrations with WADA. When he'd finished, he had expected Mary Helen to tell him he was mad but instead she issued a pep talk. Perhaps this was what he was supposed to do in life. When the time came, he should push on.

Apart from that chat, Vitaly and Yuliya's project with WADA and Robertson had pretty much gone into mothballs since Istanbul. Robertson was handcuffed, it seemed, by the same rules as the people who had introduced him to the scenario. Then the month after they'd arrived home, everything changed. Robertson, who had been friendly and solicitous via email all through the pregnancy, was back on the case in earnest. In March he emailed Vitaly with a novel proposal.

'Vitaly, I wanted to ask if you & Julie [sic] would be willing to speak with a trusted journalist? He is someone I have dealt with for about two years & I trust him. He is quite well known. He was the journalist who first broke the story about the Kenyan runners using EPO in reported large numbers & he recently broke the story about the Russian scientist selling Full Size MFG. He does impactful stories & at times has a further reach than I do in uncovering the truth. I did not give him your or Julie's name, but I mentioned I have some people within Russian sport who may be willing to talk to him confidentially. This is the two of you & others. You & Julie can remain anonymous. I have found this journalist to be credible & very caring about truth finding. He could meet you outside of Russia, & if you felt more comfortable, I could be at this meeting as well. Please let me know as soon as possible. Remember, this can be done confidentially & anonymously.'

Vitaly was in the apartment when he'd picked up the email.

'Are you serious, Jack?' Vitaly muttered before conceding to himself that Jack was nothing if not a serious man. Yes, Vitaly was willing. Thank you, Jack.

In their bedroom later that night, he floated the idea to Yuliya. Robert was sound asleep in his cot. Vitaly braced himself. He'd known better than to go running straight to her, breathlessly excited and clutching a printout of the email. This was going to be a hard sell.

'Vitaly, we've been through this before. And nothing happened. We agreed to leave it but now, three weeks later, you're on about this again? You want to speak to a journalist and do what? Be an idiot in the media?'

A year had passed since she'd supplied long chapter and detailed verse on Russian doping to WADA. One year and nothing. Point proven, she felt. Months after her letter, on the eve of the World Championships in Moscow, the *Sunday Times* of London had produced a story on Grigory Rodchenkov and how doping in Russia was being covered up. No investigation followed. Nothing. No one spoke to Vitaly about it. Nobody was interested. Point proven again and again.

'Think about it,' Yuliya said. 'Four years of communicating with WADA and nothing happens. How is talking to a journalist going to help?'

Vitaly found himself agreeing with his wife. Yet there had always been a side to Vitaly that distrusted certainty. A voice inside his head kept telling him that if you want to make God smile, you just tell him your plans. After Robert's arrival, the plan was to close the door on anti-doping. For ever. God must have really smiled when he heard that. There was, though, a corollary to making the Man Above smile: if you want to make Yuliya mad, tell her Vitaly's plans.

Over the following day, Vitaly couldn't free his brain of Jack's email. He'd tried a lot of doors that led nowhere but, for argument's sake, just suppose this next door was the one. Suppose speaking with this journalist was the door that led him where he needed to go. If he didn't open the door, he would never know. He spoke to Yuliya again. Took a different tack this time.

. 'I took this path in 2008 and I convinced you in the end to join me. It hasn't gone well, but this is another sign that we should keep trying.'

'You're still stupid, Vitaly.'

But she was worn down by his dog-with-a-bone persistence. A few days later they were being introduced to a journalist online. Jack trumpeted the introduction as if heralding the arrival of a distinguished noble to the court of Stepanov.

> 'I would like to introduce Hajo Seppelt, who is a well-respected anti-doping journalist and has experience with allegations of doping within Russia. I have known & met with Hajo & have the utmost respect for him & his work. His concern is finding &, when necessary, revealing the truth. If you choose to remain anonymous, he will honour this. I will leave it up to all of you to discuss when & where to meet. If my schedule allows me, I will join you at this meeting.'

Fortunately, Hajo Seppelt's light was not hidden under any bushels. A quick Google search revealed a solid record of documentary work on the doping issue stretching back to the late 1990s. Swimming, cycling, winter sports, North Korea even. His shelf had as many awards as his passport had stamps. And he was keen.

Vitaly and Yuliya were planning to travel to Kislovodsk in mid-April. The city was 800–1,200 metres above sea level and its hilly parklands made it popular with Russian runners at that time of year. They were intending a five-week training trip, a pleasant way for Yuliya to dip her toes back into the scene. Could they speak with Hajo when they got back?

'No,' Hajo Seppelt said, 'I will come to see you in Moscow before then.'

'Oh? Well, okay!'

This was new. Nobody Vitaly had dealt with had ever expressed urgency before, but this Hajo Seppelt had a different metabolism. He didn't tiptoe his way into your life, he burst upon it. After four years of WADA's foot-dragging, Vitaly liked that. He liked Seppelt's exuberance but also worried a little about it. Seppelt was well known as a journalist covering the anti-doping world. It was no secret that Russia closely followed the activities of prominent domestic and international journalists while their assignments concerned Russia. Sometimes these journalists just died or disappeared. Seppelt was undeterred when Vitaly mentioned his concerns.

'I've been in Moscow twice in the past couple of months. Just give me the directions to your apartment, if you think that would be the most convenient place to meet.'

Chapter 27

Hajo Seppelt brought his elemental energy to Vitaly and Yuliya's little apartment, just a couple of metro stops from Moscow's Red Square. Meetings and greetings. Tea offered and accepted. Business on the agenda. Vitaly did most of the talking. Yuliya was still tentative with her English and a tad sceptical about this latest development.

'How could a journalist achieve more than WADA?'

'Yuliya,' Vitaly said, 'when you switched sides you got on the train with me. That train is still going and you can't get off. Can we just see where it takes us?'

Into the carriage had walked Seppelt, who filled it with his enthusiasm and his enquiring nature. Vitaly spoke while Yuliya watchfully gauged the German's reactions to what was being said. Her Russian heart suspected it was never a good plan to get involved with a journalist. But Seppelt seemed serious and sure of himself. Unfazed by Russia. *Still*, she thought, *he's just a journalist*.

When they had talked for an hour, Robert awoke noisily from a nap, providing an intermission. Seppelt sat in the kitchen while Vitaly and Yuliya tended to their son in the bedroom. A whispered conference.

'So? What do you think?' asked Vitaly.

'Yeah, he seems okay.'

'Should we show him your statement to WADA?'

'Okay. If you want to.'

'If it interests him, we might actually get something done.'

They returned to the kitchen with Robert and the full ten pages of Yuliya's statement to WADA, then left their visitor to read in peace. Five minutes later, when Vitaly checked in on him, Seppelt was still flicking from one page to another. He seemed more like a prospector panning for nuggets than a serious student.

'This is just like the German Democratic Republic,' he said, and went back to his sifting. Then eventually: 'Good, this goes to the heart of why we are all here.'

Seppelt wanted to make a documentary film for television about doping in Russia, which he believed to be systematic and endemic. He already had some people who would speak without being identified. Would Vitaly and Yuliya consider speaking with their faces to camera as they told their story? Would they be the whistle-blowers that he felt the piece needed?

After his five years in the US, Vitaly's English was good. But 'whistle-blowers'? This was a new term. He'd been speaking to WADA for almost five years and not once had anyone mentioned this word. Now it turned out he had been whistle-blowing all the time. The problem had been that WADA didn't have a whistle-blowing programme and he had been whistle-blowing in the wind.

Seppelt explained further.

'You would be the two people who finally tell the world exactly how Russia has been cheating at sport. You'll speak from the inside.'

Vitaly and Yuliya had discussed this possibility and its consequences already. Speaking from the inside was fine. Staying on the inside afterwards was not. There was an old Soviet joke that had never lost currency: 'Of course, we Russians have freedom of speech, we just have no freedom *after* speech.'

'If we go public, we'll be in deep trouble in Russia,' said Vitaly. 'We would have to be out of the country before your programme is shown. We will need to be somewhere we can feel safe. You know how Russia works. It will probably mean the end of Yuliya's career, so I'll need to support my family. I will need to work. You will need to get us to somewhere safe and you need to get me work or bring me to somebody who can do that.'

They didn't want money. They didn't want fame. Infamy was inevitable. They were willing to expose the pervasiveness of Russian sports corruption but they knew exactly what that meant. Sporting prestige was the emperor's new clothes. The Communist Party had replaced the tsars, then the oligarchs had replaced the Party, but the populace were soothed and diverted as always by bread and circuses. Safe exile and a job for Vitaly seemed a reasonable ask when set against the risks and the sacrifices they would face. They had expected Seppelt to nod solemnly and say it would be done. Instead he said he had to tread carefully. That the ethics of rewarding sources had to be observed.

'And what about protecting sources,' Vitaly said. 'Do you have ethics for that? Is preventing sources from getting killed considered to be "rewarding" sources?'

'Look,' said Seppelt, 'make it simple. So maybe I don't show your faces on screen. We just tell the story.'

Vitaly smelt a cop-out and it went against the grain. He didn't want to be killed but he didn't want the story watered down, either.

'The detail of our story is very specific. You know that. Certain people watching will know who we are. The FSB will know seconds later. Your documentary will be weaker if we aren't on camera, and we will be in danger anyway. The conditions are the conditions. We will take the risk under those conditions. You should go back and think hard about this and then get back to us.'

Seppelt was disappointed, but what he had read was a story he had to tell. Filming this odd couple was an opportunity he had to take even if it meant moonlighting as a travel agent and job locator. He left with Yuliya's statement in his briefcase and a maelstrom inside his head. Since 2010 one of these two people had been passing sensitive and incriminating information to WADA about Russian doping. Meanwhile the other one had been doping. It was either a great documentary or a screwball comedy. Either way, he wanted to be the guy to make it. He lived for good stories. He knew he would be coming back. And he knew the answer he would be coming back with.

Afterwards, reviewing the visit, Vitaly and Yuliya agreed they had been impressed with Seppelt. They sensed everything that he brought to the table. He just needed to bring a little more. They weren't seeking star treatment, but they couldn't remain in a country that thought so little of shooting the messenger that it often didn't even bother covering its traces.[1] In the meantime, they would be in Kislovodsk for the month of May. Everybody could use that time for thinking.

While they were in Kislovodsk, Seppelt called Vitaly often. Ideas were bubbling in his head. He'd spoken to some people in America. They might find Vitaly work over there. An English-speaking destination would be best, no? And he was speaking to people in Germany. A parliamentarian with an interest in anti-doping. And an athletics chief. Vitaly was coming to the conclusion that Seppelt's enthusiasm meant the documentary might actually get made.

Their apartment in Kislovodsk was a five-minute walk from where Mariya Savinova and her husband, Alexey, were staying. They were in town to train. Alexey more so than Mariya, who was still on cruise setting after her London 2012 triumph. It was unclear if they owned or rented the apartment they were staying in. Property and cars came to successful Olympians in Russia, and Savinova said she had ended up owning three apartments in the months after London 2012. Property tied an athlete to Russia in a way that cash could not.

The couple had a dog, a bouncy Labrador named Joy. One day when Yuliya was at the dentist, Vitaly went out walking with Robert swaddled in a sling on his chest. He spotted the Olympic champion squatting down on the pavement, joylessly clearing up her dog's mess.

'You know, you are the first person in Russia I have ever seen do that.'

Savinova smiled up at him, a little embarrassed. Picking up dog dirt is not a champion's best look. They fell into step together, making the uneasy chat of hitherto nodding acquaintances forced to improvise something more meaningful. Vitaly was quite taken with Joy the Labrador. Savinova was very taken with Robert the baby. She was taking a break from serious running, she said, and for some time she had been hoping to become pregnant but so far nothing had happened. The blame for this was being placed on her diet of doping products. Maybe her hormones had been messed about too much, she said. She hoped the break would allow things to get back to normal.

It was a pleasant conversation and no surprise when a few days later Savinova texted Yuliya and asked if she would like to meet up for a walk and a chat in the same park. Dogs and babies were both welcome. They knew each other only slightly. They now shared a coach and had been to training camps together back in late 2012. By then Savinova had been crowned as the major star of Russian middle distance and Yuliya had been on the borders of a ban. Now Yuliya's life was filled with the sort of happiness that Savinova yearned for. They were happy in each other's company.

When she came back from the walk, Yuliya mentioned to Vitaly that they had spoken, among other things, about doping and its effects. Savinova had chatted about having been doped before the World Championships in Moscow in 2013. Kazarin had pushed Melnikov to allow her to take even more EPO just to make sure that she won on home turf. Bread and circuses. Savinova had been quite open about it all.

A day later Seppelt called Vitaly again. The conversation fresh in his mind, Vitaly mentioned how Yuliya had been swapping dope gossip with Savinova. The Olympic champion had spoken openly about her regime. The effect on Seppelt was like spreading catnip for a kitten.

'Vitaly, look, maybe Yuliya and Mariya Savinova could have the same conversation again? With a recorder running? How would that be? This could be the gold we're looking for.'

The gold had to be licensed, fenced off and mined. Or, in layman's terms, Yuliya would have to be convinced. Vitaly was coming to understand, though, that this German was a journalist to his core.

'When can we meet again, Vitaly?'

'Well, we're here for a few more weeks.'

'We really need to meet. To discuss things. I am going to get something for you, some special equipment so you can record in case there are interesting recordings in the future.'

'Hajo, you do know that we would have to have your equipment with us all the time? The conversations we have recorded in the past just happened. We can't make appointments to speak about doping and then show up with your equipment and pretend it's something to do with the baby. It just happens.'

When they hung up, they both understood they had entered new territory. There was something big to be unwrapped here. This was what Jack Robertson had in mind when he went matchmaking: put them together, stand back, see what happens.

A few days later, a second walk. Vitaly tagging along this time. As an item of interest, he ranked behind Robert the baby and Joy the dog, despite being better housetrained than either. The women chatted and Vitaly dawdled a few steps behind them like a dutiful member of household staff. Yuliya and Mariya were becoming friends. Unfortunately. Savinova was emerging as a genuinely nice person. In the past Vitaly had read interviews with her. She always seemed pretty decent and humble. She came from Chelyabinsk too, which was another small mark in her favour. She was a big star but not inside her own head.

When he caught up with them at one point, she was explaining to Yuliya how she had become a premium subscriber to Portugalov's doping service. Now, though, she and Alexey worked around it a little as Alexey had a good knowledge of drugs and he knew his wife's needs and limits. Alexey was well connected, it seemed. He had read a lot about doping and he had now become Savinova's main adviser.

Vitaly listened in, astounded at her frankness. He half-feared Yuliya was going to chip in with a gossipy moan that her own husband was a complete anti-doping fanatic. But Savinova continued chatting happily. You just have to work with Portugalov, she was saying, this is just how it is. You want to make sure you are covered, and he wants to get money for doing that, so you just pay him his money. Fact of life. She and Alexey were getting their information from Portugalov and also from Kazarin. They were instructed on how and when to dope, but in the end they were deciding for themselves. It was as if Russia's doping cafe offered various set meals with different prices but she and Alexey chose to order their drugs à la carte.

Vitaly liked Savinova too, and he could see that Yuliya enjoyed her company, but right there and then he wished he had a microphone and a boom pole. If only he could just walk behind them, dangling a mic over their heads, taping everything they said. It might kill their friendship but it could blow up the system. Everything Savinova had achieved was diminished by that system.

Despite the frank exchange of shop talk, Savinova and Yuliya's knowledge of each other's broader lives was still patchy. Nothing was said of America, for instance. Yuliya stuck to the story that Robert had been born in Chelyabinsk. Savinova, being from that city herself, was considering having her own baby in Chelyabinsk when she became pregnant.

'Yes, that would definitely be good,' said Yuliya reassuringly.

Afterwards, the affection they both felt for Savinova ambushed them a little.

'What if they ever want us to tape Mariya?' said Yuliya. 'I really don't know if I could. The system is one thing but really nice people are a different thing.'

Knowing the conversation that lay ahead, Vitaly said that nice people could be part of a bad system too. Nice people had their own decisions to make. But he didn't feel he was on firm ground, even in his own mind. Were they really going to do this?

Whoever fights monsters should see to it that in the process he does not become a monster.

Chapter 28

Vitaly loved Kislovodsk. Yuliya was starting to train seriously again, getting herself back in shape without overdoing anything. It was late spring and life had its sense of annual renewal. He loved running and he had always loved running here. Pounding the pathways cleared his head and calmed his soul like it always had. Living among professionals, he liked to pretend to himself that he was a professional too. Most days he would run twice, hitting a daily average of 25 kilometres.

He ran now while double-jobbing as a babysitter. He planned his runs for the times when Robert was scheduled to fall asleep. Robert was happily unaware of any schedule, but most days the synchronicity between his naps and Vitaly's runs was perfect. It needed to be. Vitaly pushed Robert's pram as he ran. Sometimes he could find somewhere convenient to leave the pram and then run in loops round it, all the time keeping an eye on his sleeping son. His favourite place to run was Bashkirskiy, a lovely kilometre-long loop, maybe 3 kilometres away from the apartment. The time it took to walk to the loop was enough to send Robert soundly to sleep.

One day he was on his usual run with Robert while Yuliya was at the apartment, resting up after training. It was raining but nothing biblical. Anyway Vitaly was an optimist and Robert's pram had a rain cover. All would be well. He had noticed that his son slept better and longer on the rainy days. The closer they got to the loop, however, the heavier the rainfall became. The smart move was to go home and take the day off. His heart, as it did so often, put up a better argument than his head. Surely no professional would allow a bit of weather and a sleeping baby to get in the way of a planned run?

The Bashkirskiy looped across the top of a hill. After a steep climb to get up there, you accessed a mostly flat kilometre loop. Even on dry days, fit runners trod gingerly on the 50-metre uphill climb. It was the easiest thing to just slip and fall. Approaching the climb, the rain got serious. There was accompanying thunder and lightning. It was days like this that drove Noah into the ark. Vitaly liked the challenge. Robert slept on, oblivious.

Looking back along the path behind him, Vitaly spotted Alexey Farnosov, Savinova's husband, with his brother Andrey. They climbed out of their car at the bottom of the climb. They stood for a moment in the tempest, glancing doubtfully up the hill, then dived back into their car. So much for the no-professional-would-be-deterred part of Vitaly's explanation for being out in the storm.

He pushed on. The steep path was a torrent now. Vitaly pushed the pram upwards at a fraction of the pace that the water and mud flowed downwards. Yuliya always said he was the most stubborn man she'd ever met, but the rain was blinding him now. Solution? Instead of pushing the pram, he switched to pulling it behind him as he toiled up the hill, bent into the elements. Three or four times as he climbed, the pram tipped perilously onto one of its sides. If it slipped from his grip it would drop down the hill like a boat sliding off the top of a giant wave. If that happened, he would rather just go straight into hiding under Seppelt's scheme than have to explain it to Yuliya. He began to grudgingly reassess his harsh view of the professionals' retreat. *What is wrong with me? I could be dry and warm.* By now, though, he had come so far that it was easier to push on to the top than to negotiate sliding down to the bottom. He kept going, one foot gingerly in front of the other, feeling for purchase.

Finally at the top, he felt the climber's triumph on Everest. *That was crazy, but I did it.* He parked the pram at the usual spot and began his run. Before he took off he whispered to Robert, 'I hope we survive this day. I'm going to run now. If by some chance you learn to talk while I am gone, say nothing to your mother about this. Please.'

With every step of his run, he tortured himself with thoughts of what would happen if, say, the wind ripped a branch from a tree and hurtled it towards his son. Or the rain dislodged the ground and swept half the summit away. He was soaked to the marrow and he reproached himself with every stride. *Stupid, stupid, stubborn man.* And then, twenty minutes into his 10k, the weather just surrendered. The rain dwindled as if somebody was adjusting the nozzle of a hose.

In that moment, Vitaly felt happier than he'd ever felt on this beloved peak. He was happy that Robert had slept through it all, happy that they had persevered. He had taken on the elements and survived. It was true: what didn't kill you, made you stronger. If only Russia didn't provide so much and so many that would kill you. He pushed Robert home towards their apartment and he knew that his life, Yuliya's life and of course Robert's life were going to be different on the hills that lay ahead.

Two weeks later, on 2 June, Vitaly and Yuliya left Kislovodsk, taking a train back to Moscow. Savinova and Alexey drove home three days later. Several times Yuliya texted her to ask if she would like to come to town and have tea and cake and baby chat at the apartment. There were good intentions on both sides but no follow-through.

Back in Moscow, and Seppelt was on the phone every day.

'I am coming to Moscow soon. We need to meet.'

Yes. Yes. Yes. Then one Saturday morning the phone rang. Seppelt again.

'I'm here. I'm near the Kremlin, near the Bolshoi theatre. I need to meet with you. Can you come here now?'

Vitaly made the short journey and they sat outside a nice restaurant in the summer sun. Seppelt had brought a Russian-speaking assistant with him, and announced that he had brought a crew to Moscow and hoped he would be recording an interview in the next couple of days.

'With who, Hajo?'

'With you and your wife.'

'Well, Hajo, it's good that you came to Moscow, but you didn't arrange anything with me.'

'I did say to you that I was coming next Saturday.'

'Yes. Next Saturday. Not this Saturday. Not just two days later. We only spoke on Thursday. On a Thursday, if you say "this Saturday" you mean in two days' time. Next Saturday is nine days' time.'

Seppelt conceded. The truth was that he was antsy and he didn't want his prize horses to bolt. But on a nice summer day while taking coffee near Red Square, it was easiest just to say, 'Look, the crew are here now anyway, so why not do something?'

Vitaly was willing to be interviewed but not to be taken for granted. The more he dealt with Seppelt, the more he liked him. No matter what, this guy was going to get this film made. Vitaly saw in him something of his own zeal, but the practicalities still had to be dealt with. Speaking on camera to Seppelt meant the end of life in Russia for Yuliya, Robert and him.

In 2006, President Putin had launched a programme of construction for hundreds of sporting facilities right across Russia.

The culmination saw Russia hosting the 2013 World Athletics Championships, the 2014 Winter Olympics and finally the football World Cup in 2018. Many billions would be spent. And then more billions. Never mind the corruption, smell the prestige. All that had been asked of Russia's Olympic athletes was that they should honour the investment in the Sochi Games by winning. Show the world that modern Russia is strong, confident and, most of all, successful. Show the local people how respected Mother Russia is in the world. Of course, the state was ready to help. The old Soviet machine had been fuelled by pills and injections for so long that the coaching infrastructure had fallen into decline without anybody noticing. Meanwhile, nutrition had become a science, technology had changed, and training methods had become more sophisticated, and no one in Russia had paid much attention to that. The new fix was the old fix. The only one that they knew and trusted. Take these, every second day for twenty-one days. And always keep some clean urine in your fridge.

Now the Stepanovs would tell the world that it was all a scam knowingly bankrolled by the bosses? They were to play their secret tapes and tell their vivid stories? They were going to expose Russia to the sanctions, sanctimony and scorn of its enemies?

'Hajo, I tell you now, all hell will break loose when this film gets shown.'

Seppelt was starting to recall that Moscow seldom worked out well as a destination for Germans. Vitaly's short list of demands grew no shorter. They had met each other's match in terms of stubbornness.

'Get us out of Russia so nothing happens to us,' Vitaly said. 'Get me a job because we enjoy eating food and sleeping indoors. Look after us so we can continue to look after Robert.'

Seppelt was at once acquiescent and impatient.

'I will arrange everything for you, everything will be ready. Anyway I just brought the crew, so ARD, the German state broadcaster, knows that I am here to record you.'

'Hajo, whatever you said to ARD, that is your problem not mine.'

The assistant, a chap maybe five years younger than Vitaly and blessed with fluency in both Russian and German, tried to intervene. Vitaly's temper frayed. Of the three people in the discussion, he was the only one with real skin in the game. If the interviews were recorded and broadcast, he and his family were in danger and he would have no leverage. For the others, life would go on as normal.

'I had a very good impression of you, Hajo,' Vitaly said, trying a new tone. 'I told you my part of the deal. Either you do your part and then we do interviews. Or you don't do your part and we don't do interviews.'

In the face of Vitaly's 'I'm not angry with you, Hajo, I'm disappointed' speech, Hajo trod water. In two or three weeks he would have them safely in Germany. Vitaly would have work. Too vague, Vitaly said. Round and round they went for an hour and half until Hajo threw up his hands.

'I guess there is nothing I can do to get your interviews this time.'

'Finally, you are listening to me, Hajo. Well done.'

A week later Hajo called Vitaly again. He was still arranging things. There was a difficulty with Schengen visas because usually when you apply for a visa, if you are Russian and you haven't had a Schengen visa before, you only get it for the period of time that you are being invited for ... but he was working on that.[1]

'Keep the faith, Vitaly.'

'Keep working, Hajo.'

Chapter 29

By the end of June everything had been arranged and they travelled to Germany together. Vitaly, Yuliya and Robert *en famille*.
Seppelt was waiting in the terminal at Berlin-Tegel airport. In
the car he asked casually if they were aware that Jack Robertson
happened to be in town. Did they want to meet him?

Of course.

The meeting was brief, but the fact of Robertson just being
in Berlin at all was in its way reassuring. For months after that,
there would be no more contact with Robertson or WADA. He
had ushered them onto the boat and introduced them to their
skipper, Herr Seppelt. He had pushed them gently from the
dock. He would be waiting at the far shore when they got there.

In Berlin, Seppelt introduced them to the German parliamentarian he had promised to deliver. The politician would
be able to help them out in some way at some point down the
line. In the meantime, this meeting was to be never mentioned.
Germans did secrets just as well as Russians.

Next Seppelt announced a new plan. He would drive them
to Regensburg, some distance north from Munich in the general direction of Nuremberg. A good area for athletes to train
in, he said. Vitaly and Yuliya nodded. They had never heard
of the place, but okay. They would be in the car for five hours
but there were apparently no good places in between for athletes to train.

On the drive, Seppelt had a captive audience and some things he needed to say to them. His bosses were telling him that he was on no account to get too close to these Russians that he was working with. 'These Russians' pointed out that they weren't asking him to adopt them. If he wanted to make his documentary, they didn't care how close he felt to them. The deal still was that certain things had to happen.

Seppelt said that, while all media organisations loved investigative journalists, very few of them ever wanted to pay for the investigations. If only they knew how difficult it was to get funding for investigations. ARD were good people but they didn't spring money in advance for stuff like this. He, Hajo, was paying their fares for this trip out of his own pocket. Did they see the good faith he was bringing to this? They did but—

Seppelt was interrupted by a call from a Christoph Kopp, a well-known athletics administrator in Germany and apparently a good man to know if you wanted things done within German athletics. Kopp could arrange a sit-down with Gerhard Janetzky, the head of the Berlin Athletics Federation. Mr Janetzky would be hiring people to work on the organisation of the European Athletics Championships that would be happening in Berlin in 2018.

Forget Regensburg! They turned back towards Berlin and Janetzky.

After a while Seppelt said that, as he was footing the bill, would they mind staying at his place for a while? He would move in with this mother and they could have his apartment. They were touched by his commitment and could see the stress it was causing him.

'No problem, Hajo. And thank you.'

After eight days in Germany, they returned to Moscow on 2 July. The Berlin committee would be up and running in October 2014 and had made an offer of work to Vitaly. They

left behind a letter that Seppelt asked them to sign for the attention of his bosses at ARD. The letter explained the dangers of
remaining in Russia after the whistle had been blown and the
needs they would have when they left. A letter to show good
intentions, he said.

Everybody they had met on this road had good intentions.
Everybody had said thank you for standing up for clean athletes. 'Thank you, Vitaly. Thank you, Yuliya.' Well, there was
a saying in Russia: you can't put 'thank you' in your pocket.

They decided to press on with their covert tapings. If a
documentary was ever to happen, it would need more than the
tootings of two whistle-blowers.

Seppelt seemed smart and trustworthy and, after four fruitless
years of emails to WADA, he was now their only hope. Whereas
WADA couldn't see the forest for the trees of their own rules,
Seppelt just saw prairies and pathways. No problem was without
a solution. They encouraged him to come to Moscow again
and this time they would film some interviews with him before
the month was out. Meanwhile, Vitaly noticed some of the old
determination returning to his wife's eyes.

~

Yuliya was with Mokhnev. It was 9 p.m. on 12 July 2014. She
had been back in Moscow for a while and she had agreed to
meet him for a quick catch-up.

They sat on a bench in Kazansky train station in
Komsomolskaya Square. He was waiting for a train south.
One of his few remaining athletes was travelling with him.
Mokhnev's tantrums over Yuliya's injury and her departure
from him were history now. They spoke plainly to each other,
as two people who had been through much together. Under
the clamour of trains and commuters, he lamented what his life
had become. His numbers were down. Athletes were leaving

him. His income was dwindling. His star was waning. He was still married. He was broken by the political chicanery back in Kursk. Mr Shaev was taking athletes away from him, he said. And that other hood, Markovchin, was forcing Mokhnev to take in runners that he didn't want to know, much less coach. Duds, each and every one of them.

He had her attention now. That pair! Surely not Kursk's clown double-act Shaev and Markovchin! She thought back to the day when Vitaly had intervened and extracted the 89,000 roubles from them that she had been owed. She had been so impressed with Vitaly that day. Liking him more and more even if she was not yet, to her knowledge, fully in love with him. Just married to him. But she'd seen something there.

And now she sat in Kazansky station, looking at the wreck of a man she'd once thought she loved, and listening to how the Dumb and Dumber of Kursk sports administration were playing him for a fool. She'd been right about Vitaly that day. She just hadn't learned to trust her instincts yet.

She looked again at Mokhnev and thought about all those years when he had played her and used her. How when she'd told him she was marrying Vitaly, the doping-tester guy, Mokhnev had nodded and shrugged, cocky about the grip he had on her through controlling her doping intake and her athletics coaching. He had thought he was the only one who could guide her out of Kursk. To a girl from Kursk, he thought he had been a limo pulling up at a ghetto kerb. *Hey, kiddo, I can take you away from all this.* Mokhnev's wife had once come to Yuliya's apartment, swinging an umbrella at Yuliya for using witchcraft to steal Mokhnev away from her. *Witchcraft? Look in the mirror, lady.* Mokhnev had laughed it all off and done nothing. Always cocky.

Yuliya, girl, she asked herself now, *whatever were you thinking?*

~

In the biggest country on earth, finding a location to do some filming was a problem. Public spaces were out of the question. Igor and Olga still shared the apartment, and relations showed no sign of improving. Finally, they settled on a system of listening in on their flatmates' conversations in the apartment to ascertain when they would be gone for a few hours. As soon as they were out of sight, the German film crew were ushered in. The arrangement provided a dramatic tension. What if Igor and Olga returned unexpectedly? 'Guys, this is not how it looks!' Yuliya did one interview in Seppelt's hotel room, but it was so cramped that it was difficult to disguise the specific location.

It surprised Vitaly and Yuliya how many hours of interview were committed to tape for a one-hour documentary. Hopefully Seppelt hadn't blown the budget for editing. Otherwise they were comfortable with the process. And keen to deliver for Seppelt.

Yuliya suggested that, if he could stall things until November, they might bring him tapes from the training camp in Kyrgyzstan. They would be there with Kazarin and some prominent athletes. Seppelt had the fidgety metabolism of a deadline journalist, though. Sit on a hot story for any length of time and your life disappears into a swamp of what-ifs. The journalist in him wanted to press on. Another voice was in his ear, however. Somebody counselling caution.

Jack Robertson had often told him to make haste slowly. The same Jack Robertson had been doing some thinking. Since its inception, the WADA code had been governed by two editions of its own accord. The 2004 version was superseded by a second code on 1 January 2009. WADA moved at a snail's pace, but in November 2011 it had begun drafting a third code for itself. This had been ratified in Johannesburg in 2013. With a few i's dotted and several t's crossed, the third WADA code would come into effect on 1 January 2015.

The relevance to Seppelt was that, after that date, WADA would no longer need to ask individual countries to investigate themselves. The world's anti-doping police would at last have the power to establish their own independent investigations. If Seppelt's piece aired months before the advent of the new code, his work would most likely be swept under the same carpet that concealed Vitaly's email correspondence with WADA. Public-relations experts would appear as if by magic to perfume the room with soothing scents. The effort and risk would be wasted. By contrast, if the documentary landed on screens on a date close to early January 2015, WADA would have the opportunity to show that it had recently acquired some backbone and the muscles to go with it. Russia wasn't a bad place to start flexing those muscles. In fact, it would be embarrassing if WADA failed to do just that. Checkmate!

When Robertson had set up the first blind date with Seppelt, Vitaly and Yuliya hadn't sensed the wisdom in his matchmaking. Now they were beginning to think they had underestimated Robertson. Wisdom? More like genius.

~

Kazansky station. Mokhnev was still talking about Kursk and the car crash that his life had become. Yuliya's mind slipped back to the evening when she had finally left him. She had gone to see Mokhnev after speaking with Kazarin about being trained by him. Mokhnev sensed that it was the end. That his hold over her was gone. His cockiness shrivelled. He became angry. Really angry. Not like when she had announced her intention to marry. He shouted at her that she was a traitor. She didn't care. She was free. If only Mokhnev knew the whole story. He had been so sure of himself. He had encouraged her to marry

Vitaly. Laughing at her. Playing his long game. Now Vitaly had encouraged her to join Kazarin and it was all over for Mokhnev. Mistress gone. Meal ticket gone. He was now just small change from Kursk.

On the bench in Kazansky station now, he boasted pathetically about a little earner he had going down, across the border in Ukraine. He had made 5,000 roubles the other day.

'Does your wife know you are earning a bit extra?' Yuliya asked, puncturing him.

'She doesn't know where I am.'

He still had a trace of the old bravado. Just nothing to back it up.

'Are things really bad for you financially?'

'Why should they be bad? Why not make a bit on the side? I left the trials yesterday and went away for a while. Where, for crying out loud, can you earn five thousand these days?'

She tuned in and out of his litany of woes. This athlete ruined by another coach giving her shots since she was seventeen, another was too heavy, that one is too lazy, and all the others are running off to other coaches. He spoke about one of his athletes leaving the team. Another low blow.

'Well, why is *she* leaving you?'

'I don't know why. I don't give her any pharma. And her attitude. If only she trained. But all she does is fuck everything that moves. If she hasn't got her claws into one, then it'll be another or even a third. I just don't want to spend as much money on her as I'm spending on Kupina. I need her like a hole in the head.'

Yekaterina Kupina was another 800 metres runner. When Yuliya had become injured and stopped being a prospect for London, she had noticed the increased attention Mokhnev lavished on Kupina, who had arrived in his training group that summer. Kupina was six months older than Yuliya but she was the new prospect. Early twenties and, sure enough, in the seasons of 2012 and 2013 she had produced her best stuff. Yuliya knew the magic behind those improved times. She almost felt sorry for the girl.

Mokhnev yammered on. When Kupina had been on Parabolan last summer, the 2013 season, she had passed a doping control test on the fifteenth day. The fifteenth day after her last dose! Others needed to be 'clean' for twenty-one days before their doping control. Miracles happen! Next came the inevitable boast: Mokhnev admittedly had paid 7,000 roubles to steer Kupina's sample safely through the test. Still, not a lot of money. He had been amazed and surprised when the all-clear came.

Keep talking, thought Yuliya. She resisted the urge to glance down at her phone. *Keep talking. I always knew your big mouth would finish you.*

He rambled on. Some bizarre story now about swapping a minibus for a talented young athlete.

'What?'

'I said, "If you've been giving her injections, if she's ruined by you, then you return me the bus after a year ..." He said, "And how will you find out?" And I said, "Because I won't do anything."'

'She won't run,' Yuliya said, knowing his mind.

'Maybe she won't run,' Mokhnev said. 'And that will be that.'

Wherever all this was leading, all this taping and dealing with WADA and Seppelt, she had known for some time that there was no going back. And now, listening to Mokhnev in Kazansky station, she was happy about that. Happy inside. Doors were slamming behind her. Finally, she was making good choices.

~

The summer in Moscow was happy and productive. Robert was a joy, and Vitaly and Yuliya made efforts to patch up relations with Igor and Olga. Yuliya trained regularly with her friends in the city. Vitaly stole enough time for his own runs. They competed for fun in small summer competitions around Moscow, happy unofficial gatherings. They wheeled Robert along in his pram to be fussed over while they ran races and gossiped with friends. They were doing what they enjoyed doing and the days were cloudless. The season was passing too quickly.

There was a relay race scheduled for the middle of August, a novel event. Teams of four made up of two women and two men would compete. They asked Igor and Olga if they would make up a team just for the fun of it. The boys ran 400 metres legs and the girls ran 200 metres legs. Twenty teams. Heats, semis and a final. They came third and loved it. For one splendid late-summer evening they all had fun together.

This was running as Vitaly always imagined it. He was on a roll. Sunday 31 August was the day of days. Nike had organised a small competition. As a promotion you could try on a pair of Nike's new shoes and even run a race in them. If you won a race wearing the blue Nike Pegasus shoes you were trying out, you got to take them home with you. Even Vitaly, an old-school Corinthian at heart, was a little pumped. But Yuliya's actual participation in the 1000 metres race for women was a source of angst between them.

'Yuliya, I don't think you should be in it.'

'Don't be ridiculous. No one here cares. It's a fun thing.'

'But you're banned and you're also an elite-level athlete.'

'You're really taking this too seriously.'

She tried to laugh it off, to get him to lighten up on this one and laugh with her. He wouldn't budge.

'The Pegasus shoes mightn't mean much to you, but they would to a lot of other runners in your race. You're robbing them of the opportunity.'

This guy, she thought, *you can't win with him.* Sometimes it was better to let him win the argument and do what you were going to do anyway. She wanted to feel that thrill again, the power in her legs. So she raced and she cruised to victory and the Pegasus shoes were hers. Only her husband could forbear to cheer.

Vitaly himself qualified for the finals of both the 1000 metres and the 800 metres races. He opted for the 800 metres as he was the only man in the world whose lucky number was 800. Also there was a guy in 1000 metres who was so good that he would probably lap Vitaly.

In the final, the three favourites were disconcertingly young. Vitaly asked one whippersnapper what his personal best was, and was told 2:02. Vitaly thought he could take him. That was just last month, the young fellow added. Then, just before the race, Vitaly spotted the same kid changing into a pair of Nike spikes. Everybody else was wearing the promotional blue Nike Pegasus shoes. Wearing them and getting to keep them if you won was half the fun. But the young guy was choosing his own spikes.

'You don't need the Nike sneakers?'

'Nah, I have about ten pairs of them at home.'

Screw you, Vitaly thought. *This race is the classic wily veteran (me) in sneakers against the arrogant spoiled tyro (you) in spikes. Bring it on.*

The first lap was slow. Vitaly lolloped around in last place, waiting. The track was only 333 metres around so it wasn't the standard two-lap deal for an 800 metres race. *The surface is annoyingly suitable for spikes*, thought Vitaly as they came around the bend. He would have to make his move soon. There was still no sign of the young guy breaking for glory.

Vitaly was too old to prosper in a helter-skelter finish so, calculating that the race had 400 metres left, he moved through the field, surprising them before he even found top gear. Not that he wanted to find top gear too early. He wouldn't have the fuel to sustain it to the finish. Sure enough, with 200 metres left, the young spikes guy passed him like a train.

Shit, Vitaly thought, *all I have been doing is making the pace for him.*

The kid was 5 metres clear with 50 metres to go. Cruising. Winning and showing everybody that he was used to the feeling. Coming onto the straight, Vitaly spotted Yuliya running alongside the track, 15 or 20 metres ahead of him. She had Robert in his pram, animated like he'd never seen her, shaking her fist and screaming.

'Come on, Vitaly. Come on!'

It was the most beautiful thing he had ever seen. He was in cinematic slow motion now, feeling every lengthening of his stride as the theme music from *Chariots of Fire* pulled him home. She was running alongside him, pushing their son along, screaming for him to succeed. Yuliya and his son.

The spikes kid's back loomed close enough to touch. Just 20 metres to go. Vitaly couldn't even feel his own legs. Were his feet even striking the track? It was the greatest feeling in the world. Just 10 metres now and they were shoulder to shoulder. *What have you got, spikes boy?*

Vitaly crossed the line, half a metre ahead.

Hey, Mokhnev! Hey, Melnikov! Hey, Portugalov! Wish you were here! You haven't sucked all the joy out of this world. Not yet. I wish you were here to see this. Really I do.

They passed the rest of the evening walking together in the evening sun, taking in the remaining races. One man, his wife, his new son and his new blue Nike Pegasus shoes. Bliss.

Towards the end of the evening, Nike put out a whisper that there soon would be a famous guest among them. It was true. Mariya Savinova, Alexey and Joy the dog turned up just to wave and to be waved at. Yuliya and Vitaly spent a while making small talk with the celebrity guests. Vitaly wondered uncharitably if the kid with ten pairs of Nikes under his bed might ask for a selfie with the Stepanov family and their friends.

Chapter 30

In the autumn the hotline to Hajo Seppelt went quiet. A free-lance journalist's career needs a steady flow of pay cheques, and Seppelt was busy elsewhere, delving into the eternally murky world of cycling. For the time being, Vitaly and Yuliya flew down to Chelyabinsk with Robert.

Time had passed quickly since Yuliya had sat in an office listening to Melnikov and Kazarin tell her how much they themselves were suffering due to her imminent ban. Recently Kazarin had called to tell Yuliya that, with the end of her ban now in sight, he had arranged a tie-up for her with his club, Nizhny Tagil, near Yekaterinburg. When the ban ended in a few months' time, Yuliya would be hired again. Yekaterinburg was the most important city in the region, bigger and more influential than Chelyabinsk.

Kazarin managed to make Yuliya's reinstatement as a paid member of the Nizhny Tagil club sound like an immense favour that he was in a position to bestow. She recalled his promise two years ago that her club membership and her income would not be affected if she accepted her ban without fuss or appeal. He had forgotten those words, it seemed. Now he was making a big deal out of what he had already promised but failed to deliver. He had also said that, not only would she train with the club through her ban, but that she would also be back at her best the moment the ban ended and that she would go on to win a medal in Rio.

'Don't worry about the ban,' he'd said, 'you just sign the papers.'

Just a few weeks later the director of the Nizhny Tagil club had called Yuliya.

'As was promised to you, I am not going to fire you but, just in case somebody asks questions, you do need to write me a resignation letter. Just to be on the safe side. Just in case there is a check. At least I can show that you were fired because you are a doper. I will keep paying you, don't worry.'

That was March 2013. Yuliya wrote the letter. No more salary ever appeared. When Kazarin triumphantly announced that he was plugging her back into the system, Yuliya examined the new phone she had bought to check out the recording function.

For a change they had flown to Chelyabinsk this time as the road trips had become wearying. They left Robert with Vitaly's parents while they drove to Nizhny Tagil in Vitaly's dad's car. They broke the journey for a brief meeting with Kazarin himself. He needed a favour. Could they drop documents to the club, which was a full hour-and-a-half drive further up the road from where he lived? When he pulled up for the handover, Kazarin was behind the wheel of a sleek Mercedes S-Class vehicle. Not doing too badly for a humble Russian athletics coach.

'On your way back,' he insisted, 'you guys really must drop into my apartment.'

In Nizhny Tagil they met with the club director. Yuliya taped the conversation but the issue of doping never came up. She didn't even ask what had happened to the wages she had been promised.

When they found Kazarin's apartment on the way back, the plan was for Vitaly to remain in the car while Yuliya spoke to her coach and taped him. He was unlikely to hold forth on doping matters if Vitaly was within earshot. Yet Yuliya returned to the car just five minutes after she had left it.

'He insists that you come in to join us.'

Their evening with Kazarin was interesting and bizarre. Early on, Kazarin showed them a pin that he had been given by the police club, Dinamo.

'The highest honour the police can give,' he boasted. 'This is gold and these are diamonds. Twenty thousand euros' worth.'

That Mercedes. This gold pin. The very apartment they were sitting in. He was so pleased. He was the coach of both the gold medallist and the bronze medallist at the Olympics. There would be more of all this for him. Forget the past, he seemed to be saying, just follow me and you could have all this as well.

They ate with Kazarin and his wife. The talk touched on doping only peripherally. Kazarin spoke about preparation and said that Yuliya would have to take it slow this year. Just vitamins and nothing else. Whether this conservative approach was for Vitaly's benefit or not was hard to know, but it seemed wise. A second ban would be for a lifetime, and Kazarin and his colleagues would have to be very sure of the lie of the land before they began exposing real prospects to lifetime bans. It had been a wasted evening and it was late when they got back to Chelyabinsk. Vitaly's parents, unfamiliar with the design of the modern nappy, had been putting Robert's nappies on the wrong way around all day. Robert had survived the indignity, though.

In mid-September they left Chelyabinsk and returned to Moscow for a few weeks. The apartment was too small for the two couples. They chafed. The addition of a small baby caused the atmosphere to overheat. One evening Igor snapped. Robert was a little animal, he said, and if he saw the little animal on the kitchen floor again he was going to kick him.

That was that. The summer truce snapped. The lull was over. Yuliya said flatly that she would not speak to Igor again. Ever. She left with Vitaly and Robert for a training camp in

Kislovodsk on 10 October. They would be gone for twenty-one days and everybody was relieved to have some space.

They had decided to intensify their efforts to gather the evidence of Russia's pathological cheating. If Seppelt's film was to trigger a WADA investigation, they would need to furnish him with sustainable proof. Hearsay and good anecdotes wouldn't cut it. Yuliya had taped Mokhnev's foolish gabblings in Moscow. In Kislovodsk Yuliya now added two more recordings to the catalogue. Ekaterina Poistogova, the bronze medallist in the 800 metres at London 2012, made a weighty contribution to her own comeuppance when she chatted about how she intended to get herself ready for the summer season with a course of ten oxandrolone pills.

'Why not take more, Ekaterina?'

'Well, they take three months to clear the system. You know that?'

Obligingly she chattered freely about her adventures with EPO.

Replaying the tapes later gave them a shiver. After years of Russia's brazen cheating, its athletes were casually condemning themselves out of their own mouths. The culture had become so pervasive that talking openly about doping wasn't even a taboo. They showcased their knowledge in conversations. They advised and admonished others. There was a knowing swagger to their cheating.

Meanwhile, Seppelt was back in business. While they were in Kislovodsk, he was beginning work on a cut of his documentary. Every night he would call them with requests. Information. Transcripts. Advice. Ideas. He nudged Vitaly to scan through the recordings of Melnikov and Kazarin from back in early 2013 to see what, if anything, might be of use. If there were more recordings to come, he was interested too. He said that he hoped to present Vitaly and Yuliya as a couple of vulnerable young truth-tellers who felt so threatened that they had to flee Russia.

The truth-tellers themselves weren't so keen on this dramatic angle. Certainly they would be leaving Russia and they understood that when the documentary screened they would be under serious threat. But they didn't see it as helpful to make their human situation the cornerstone of the documentary. The message was about the doping. Not about the messengers.

Events lent momentum to the project.

Yuliya had become zealous in her conversion. The system that had once promised to cradle her, she now saw as a heartless exploitation factory. When you offered the system something, you received love, rewards and drugs. When your stupid human needs outstripped your potential, the system spat you out. She felt foolish. How often had she told Vitaly he was a gullible fool, that she alone knew how the real world worked? She decided she would make better recordings when they went to Kyrgyzstan. Seppelt was still pressing for more and she would deliver something that showed the full extent of the Russian system. By doing so, she would break any chains that connected her to it.

There was a ten-day gap between the training camps in Kislovodsk and Kyrgyzstan, and lots to do. Robert was fast approaching his first birthday. They would be in Kyrgyzstan on the day of his celebrations, so they needed to fit all his one-year appointments with Moscow's doctors and paediatricians into the ten-day window.

Seppelt was pushing hard for them to spend the ten-day gap time in Berlin. It didn't suit Vitaly and Yuliya to travel to Germany, but being caged in Moscow with Igor and Olga didn't suit them either. So Yuliya told her training group that she would be in Moscow, taking care of Robert. Vitaly told his parents that they were going to Kursk. They travelled from Kislovodsk back to Moscow and flew straight to Berlin early the next morning. In Berlin, Vitaly worked with Seppelt, sifting and editing footage. Yuliya trained when she could and took care of Robert in her free hours. There was an interesting and vibrant city out there, but they weren't going to see it this time.

On 8 November they returned to Moscow. They had just five hours in the city before boarding a plane at Domodedovo. Five hours from airport to apartment and back to airport, having changed and packed. Mercifully those five hours began at midnight, when the Moscow traffic merely slowed their taxi rather than bringing it to a standstill.

It took six more hours to fly to Manas International airport near Bishkek, the capital of Kyrgyzstan. Their destination, the training camp at Lake Issyk-Kul, was still a five-hour drive away on bad roads. Outside it was cold. Many minus-degrees of cold. Heavy snow was in the air, and in the distance the mountains were already coated white. Before the drive they had to wait some more. The main training party was travelling as a group from Yekaterinburg. For twelve long hours they sat in the warmth of the airport with Robert. Whipped by fatigue, they became giddy. A policeman accosted Vitaly for laughing loudly.

'Are you drunk?'

'No. Is it illegal here to laugh?'

'Maybe.'

When the belching bus disgorged everybody, it was past 5 a.m. They had been on the go with Robert for the guts of two days. Now they were billeted at the Kapriz Hotel in the little village of Baktuu-Dolonotu. Kazarin surprised Vitaly and Yuliya with the consideration he had put into securing their accommodation. Instead of the standard room, they had been given a junior suite with a bedroom and lounge on the first floor at the front of the hotel. It made being at training camp with a one-year-old toddler a little bit easier.

The Kapriz was a perfect spot for runners. It was a modern hotel dropped down sensitively in the middle of a nature reserve and surrounded by beautiful, unspoiled woods. The great lake glistened a hundred metres or so down from the hotel building. There was a spa and a swimming pool and the patchiest of Wi-Fi services.

The lake itself had once been part of the Silk Road, and there was a strand of academic which thought that the Black Death had originated and spread from here. Apart from the rough beauty of the place, this was its claim to fame. Destroyer of one-third of Europe's population. Later the lake was a torpedo-testing site for the Soviet navy and as such it had been closed to foreigners for a long time. At 663 metres deep at the middle, the water sat like a dark eye in the swollen lid of the Tian Shan mountains. The mountains were bare and in the evening sun they sat golden and mythical. The peaks were capped in snow for as far as the eye could see.

The whole area was re-establishing itself as a holiday resort, at least for the summer months. It had everything to offer the world except proximity to the world. For Russian athletes, though, it was tailor-made for training and would have been so even had the plague still lingered. It took three or four days for the body to adapt to the altitude but, when it had, there were picturesque places to run and decent places to stay and, best of all, even the most fanatical doping control officer couldn't muster the enthusiasm for the journey to get there. The athletes who came here could work hard and feel safe. As such, the trips to Kyrgyzstan were always an opportunity for coaches to dole out the drugs and paraphernalia for the forthcoming season. At Lake Issyk-Kul every athlete was handed their drugs and advised to store them in containers labelled with brand names like Nurofen or Ibuprom. Beyond that, if they got caught at the airport, any explanations as to the contents were the athlete's own problem.

Vitaly and Yuliya grabbed a few hours of sleep and went

down to lunch in the dining area. It was a Russian national team training camp so the food was good. They checked in with Kazarin, who asked Yuliya if she would call by his room later in the day for a chat. He had vitamins for her, he said, a diplomatic evasion made out of respect to Vitaly's presence.

They already had two tapes of Kazarin in the bag. One they had recorded in the office with Melnikov that first afternoon, which seemed so long ago now. The other recording was from the National Indoors a short while later. Kazarin was a national coach, though, and seemed to be about to do a U-turn on his recent enlightened suggestion that Yuliya might remain drug-free for a while. If he was going to dole out drugs in his room later, Yuliya wasn't going to pass up the audio-visual opportunity on offer.

It was shortly after 8 p.m. when Yuliya knocked on Kazarin's door. With her phone, she walked into these meetings feeling like a spy. Inside she felt nervous but it didn't show. Every new recording felt the most nerve-racking, but she played it as Vitaly thought she should. Don't try to hide the phone, leave it in the most obvious and visible place. Pick it up if that feels natural. But this was Kazarin, one of the big fish, who was maybe going to slip the noose around his own neck. That brought extra excitement and more fear. Until this point, she had been running heats without incident. Now this was a final and anything could happen. There was going to be a transfer of steroids from the coach of Russia's Olympic gold and bronze 800 metres medallists to an athlete. The athlete was going to record it all in audio and on video.

Vitaly had rehearsed it all. Audio taping was easy. The screen remained blank and the phone just did its work. If the worst came to the worst and somebody drew attention to her device, she had mentally rehearsed her routine. She would express surprise. She'd wonder aloud as to precisely what the phone was doing. She'd switch it off and shake her head at it. *Technology. It really does have a mind of its own. I'm such a clueless blonde!*

Still she was nervous. They were a long, long way from Moscow. A long, long way even from the nearest airport. Life could get extremely unpleasant extremely quickly if these people worked out what was happening. Vitaly and Yuliya had developed the habit of telling so many lies about where they were at any given time that they scarcely knew themselves if they were now where they had said they'd be. It would be a long time before they were missed if anything happened.

Yuliya was using two phones. One she would hold in her hand and the other she would place in her bag. Both phones had covers over their screen. Their technology wasn't comparable with anything from a Bond movie but she and Vitaly had become a little bit more sophisticated in their weaponry. Vitaly had installed new software whereby Yuliya could start recording on video and, with the screen covered, nobody could detect any sign that her phone had sprung to life. Again, if there was any hint of suspicion indicated, she would express bafflement and pick up the phone to examine it, pressing the off button as she did so. Anyway it seemed more odd not to carry a mobile phone than to be constantly fidgeting with one. Robert was with her at the camp and she needed to be contactable in case of emergency.

Kazarin said he was torn. That his heart told him he shouldn't be starting Yuliya on a course of pharma right now when her current ban hadn't even expired. It was madness. He had agreed with Melnikov back in Moscow that, yes, it was best to wait. But, well, his head said to get her going again. When she was free to compete once more, she could blow the field away from day one. Yuliya didn't want to sound too eager. She was still banned and another positive would finish her career. She needed evidence, not the pills. But the evidence was the pills.

'Do you think should we prepare for winter or should we wait?' he mused.

'I don't know. What do you say?'

'With the preparations?'

'What do you say?'

'Yes, I'm, like, having my doubts, you see. As if—'

'Doubts?'

'I'm thinking, are we not a bit early? In the sense that maybe it should be left for the winter. Or . . . do you need support?'

'Well, it probably wouldn't do any harm. So that I wouldn't be the weakest in the group.'

She switched the discussion to focus on what she had done under previous coaches. All doping coaches were peacocks and they liked to display a plumage more impressive than their rivals. She said that she had previously used pills, EPO and testosterone. On cue, Kazarin said he wasn't impressed about the testosterone. He was more of an EPO man. Yuliya enquired about HGH.

'But . . . is there human growth hormone? Is it still undetectable, do you know?'

'Well, they are also already saying that it can be detected. Well, to be honest, I tried them. I also don't see any—'

'There aren't any, yeah?'

'Particular effects. Yes . . . Like, it costs quite a lot, but there aren't any particular effects. Therefore we're left with oxandrolone, Primobolan.'

'Uh huh.'

'That is why we only have oxandrolone and Primobolan and, at some point in the early stages, just a little, you can do a few ampoules of EPO, of course. But make sure there are no checks at the time, nothing like that, to make sure you don't move out of the corridor.'

The 'corridor' was slang for the parameters within which athletes' ABP blood levels were tested. If you stayed within the upper and lower limits you were safely within the corridor. At certain times and places you could be outside the corridor, but otherwise it was wisest to stay within it.

She mentioned Portugalov. Kazarin seemed to regard Portugalov as a rival rather than a guru. He was reluctant to use Portugalov, he said because 'he forgets everything'.

Surprised to find a crack in the wall, she pursued this.

'Probably because he has too many people,' said Kazarin. 'When I was visiting him, he had people from swimming – coaches and athletes, other kinds of sport, cross-country skiers. He has too many people and so is apparently forgetting things.'

'Well, that is why we do it . . . without him.'

It was time to get back to the point. Enough talking about what was available elsewhere.

'Well,' said Kazarin, 'what are we going to do?'

'We're going to prepare ourselves.'

'Well, okay, then I'll give you ten tablets now. You take them.'

'Uh huh.'

'Probably, some time from Wednesday.'

Wednesday was 12 November. She had a question.

'So it works out before the 22nd?'

'Before the 22nd, yes. There are 10 milligrams each there. Here. Then, before the sample, nothing else is needed.'

'Good.'

Camp was ending on 1 December. Kazarin said that if she finished taking the tablets on 22 November it would take forty to forty-five days for them to be excreted naturally from her system.

'That means that by around the beginning of January you'll already be clean.'

This was a comfortable margin of safety, he felt. In fact, it was so comfortable that he reconsidered and decided to give her fifteen tablets. Take them till the 27 November. Be clean by 10

January. She expressed her admiration for his genius. She would have to take tests to be reinstated but meanwhile there was a margin to be exploited. He asked if she needed any syringes. Well, yes. Why not?

Sitting opposite her across a small coffee table, he put the pills on the table and asked her to count them. As she did so, he went to the closet where he'd fetched the pills from. She had been holding her phone casually, capturing glimpses of him in and out of focus, but too nervous to point the device straight at him. When he went to the closet, however, she let the phone sweep over the tablets.

Beep. Beep. Beep.

What the fuck? Fuck!

He turned around quickly. His eyes sweeping the room. She looked at him. Frozen.

'Ah,' he says. It was his phone. It was ringing.

Her heart started beating again.

Kazarin spoke into his phone. An athletics official had arrived in the hotel and he would have to go down to the dining area for a meeting. Yuliya rose to leave and gathered everything up. At the door she turned back to Kazarin.

'Righto, thank you for all the sweeties.'

'Go on.'

As planned, she kept the camera running for the minute it took her to move from the third floor down to their suite on the first. She came into their room, still filming what she was carrying, and laid the stash on the table.

'1, 2, 3, 4, 5, 6, 7, 8, 9, 10, 11, 12, 13, 14, 15. Fifteen tablets. That's all that the coach gave me. Fifteen tablets of oxandrolone. I have to take them between 12 November and 27 November. Place them under the tongue. One tablet a day. They leave the system after forty to forty-five days. On 10 January I should be clean.'

Aaaaaand CUT!

She was drained but she knew that now there would be no room for anybody to ask if this footage had been cut and spliced. It was continuous.

When they checked the phone later there was a brief and usable shot of Kazarin passing the gear over. It was short in duration and slightly out of focus but for a rookie director Vitaly's plan had worked well. They went to sleep knowing that they had got the most important recording yet, the quality of evidence that they had been promising Seppelt for months. This was stuff worth waiting for. And there would be more.

Vitaly was going to need an internet cafe. The Wi-Fi at the Kapriz was so patchy that strapping a memory stick to the ankle of a pigeon and flinging it out the window towards Berlin would be as reliable a form of transfer. From the hotel to Cholpon-Ata was 5 kilometres on foot or fifteen minutes in a taxi. Cholpon-Ata was the only decent-sized town in the region and the only place with an internet cafe, albeit one with an extortionate tariff system. Every minute spent transmitting videos and tapes to Seppelt brought Vitaly closer to bankruptcy. It could take an hour and a half to get the 'rushes' across to Seppelt in Berlin. If the connection died, Vitaly had to begin again. It was stressful. But, returning by taxi, he strolled into the lobby like a man who had just been taking the mountain air while his wife and baby napped.

Every day Yuliya was making more recordings. On every group training run that she was a part of, she recorded the chit-chat. She would return and provide a summary of what had been discussed. Then, after a quick lunch, Vitaly would head to Cholpon-Ata. There was such a volume of material coming to Seppelt every day that he chanced his arm and asked Vitaly if he could provide transcripts too. It would make the good stuff easier to locate. If Seppelt had poked his head out his window in Berlin, he might have heard the howls of frustration from the shore of Lake Issyk-Kul.

It was a difficult time. Yuliya was being pushed at training. She had worked reasonably hard during her time away, but this was a step up. Between that and the stress of making daily tapes and looking after Robert, her patience threshold was low. An athlete just wants to train, eat, rest and see the physio. Instead she was moonlighting as an undercover agent and she had her infant son in tow.

Vitaly ran once a day. Barely enough to calm him.

Seppelt had some crazy ideas. He suggested that Vitaly might leave Kyrgyzstan for three or four days, come to Berlin to do some work on the recordings and transcripts, and then fly back again. Maybe the entire family could come. He was indefatigable.

'Think, Hajo,' Vitaly said. 'Think. We're 1,600 metres above sea level. It takes four days to adjust. How is Yuliya going to explain disappearing from national training camp for four days just after she gets used to the altitude? Then she comes back and she feels sick for another four days as she adjusts again?'

'Okay,' Hajo said, 'you just come on your own, then. I'll buy the tickets.'

'It really doesn't matter. You can send a magic carpet to collect me. I'm not coming. I can't disappear. They don't like me. They'll ask questions.'

Seppelt was on edge. He had promised that his documentary would go out on 3 December. He had also inveigled Vitaly and Yuliya into attempting more recordings when they got back to Moscow. The clock wouldn't stop ticking.

Regardless, Yuliya was clear in her head about everything that needed to be done. She had a son now. Sport, as she had known it, was not what she wanted to hand on. Some days at camp the topic of doping never came up and instead they gossiped about rivals and affairs and money. On those days Yuliya would return to her room deflated, and Vitaly would just place the useless recording in a file on his laptop. Twice other athletes asked Yuliya half-jokingly why she brought her phone with her everywhere, even on runs. Robert wasn't just her son but her alibi also.

One afternoon, Yuliya came back and Vitaly asked the usual question. Any doping talk?

'Yeah, Bazdyreva!'

'Who?'

'She's new. So full of herself. And it turns out she is an expert on doping.'

Anastasiya Bazdyreva was one of Kazarin's 800 metres crew. So great was the depth of talent at that distance that it sometimes seemed as if Russia was stockpiling female 800 runners in case of a world shortage. Bazdyreva was fresh, young and full of confidence but with nothing to back it all up as yet. In Lake Issyk-Kul she was the definition of a nobody. The other runners found her loud, aggressive and not too bright. Mainly loud.

Yuliya had found herself paired with Bazdyreva on a warm-up run. Yuliya had her phone in her hand as usual and, without much expectation, she struck up some conversation. She mused about whether she should resume banned substances while still banned. Bazdyreva had just been waiting to be uncorked. Why, she was an expert on all this shit. Finally, somebody had come to her and asked. It was like those Chinese, she was saying when Yuliya tuned in, you know some kind of dragon on the Chinese steroids that everyone uses around the world.

This was unexpected. Yuliya popped her phone up a little higher as she ran, as if she needed to keep an eye on the screen for Robert-related bulletins from Vitaly.

'Sorry, you were saying?'

Bazdyreva babbled on. And on. Even when they finished

running and started stretching, her extempore lecture on doping was still in full swing. She usually ran well on Anabol, she said, as if hinting at a suitable Christmas present should Yuliya find herself in a quandary about what to get her. She spoke about Parabolan and the wash-out periods involved. She explained to Yuliya that she had stopped taking the Parabolan ninety days prior to the Russian Championships. She 'didn't have to worry'. She talked about the side effects that anabolic steroids had on others. She was lucky, she said, she never experienced the same side effects.

Yuliya had mentioned early in the conversation that Kazarin had given her drugs on the first night at the hotel. She couldn't remember what they were. Bazdyreva was alive with curiosity. Could Yuliya tell her what the packaging looked like? How did they taste? Any unusual features? If Bazdyreva got this information, she could process it in her learned mind and let Yuliya know just what she was taking and how good it was. Or not. Bazdyreva came back to those Chinese steroids. She couldn't recall the brand.[1] The ones with the dragon? You must know them, everybody takes them.

Chapter 31

Robert's first birthday fell slap in the middle of the camp, on 17 November. Another reason for Vitaly not to be marked absent without leave. Yuliya was old-fashioned about these landmarks. She felt that children should always have parties on important dates, that the stages of their lives should be recorded and celebrated. Vitaly, the man who didn't dance or drink at his own wedding, wasn't sold on the idea. Robert, he told Yuliya, wasn't going to know it was his birthday.

Vitaly's main objection was one of timing. They had planned to flee Lake Issyk-Kul on 18 November. When everybody came down for breakfast that morning, the Stepanovs would just be gone. Their tickets were already booked. The camp would continue as planned until 1 December but the Stepanovs would have vanished twelve days earlier. Did they really need to complicate matters by having a birthday party the previous day?

Yes, said Yuliya, they did. If there was a big fuss (which she still doubted there would be) when the documentary got shown, she said every athlete featured would deny that they even knew her. She had been banned for two years, hadn't she? How would they have come across her at a camp? The tapes were obviously fake, they would claim. But a birthday party was an opportunity for group photos and videos. 'Here we all are, together on the occasion of my son's first birthday just a couple of weeks ago. We're all so happy and laughing in this picture.'

And so on 17 November there was a celebration of Robert's birthday in the hotel dining room. Vitaly saw it as a little going-away do. The party was well intentioned but odd. Athletes couldn't enjoy vodka in the presence of their coaches while attending a party for a one-year-old at training camp. Besides, the group weren't teammates in the sense that would be understood in a team sport. They were self-motivated individuals who happened to train together for administrative convenience. Also, a handful of them simply didn't like or trust the Stepanovs, so they stayed away.

Some of the women made a fuss of Robert, though he had developed a temperature and was as subdued as the party itself. Vitaly hovered in the background, untroubled by people coaxing him to do otherwise, while he took a few group photos and smiled as best he could. Kazarin made a toast to Yuliya. A fine runner and one who always listened to her coaches, he said. Why, he and Melnikov had suggested to her once that she get pregnant, and within three weeks, lo, it was done.

Vashee zdaróvye! Your health!

The gathering was pleasant in its way, but any good memories were going to clear the athletes' systems long before their little blue pills did. It broke up at around 10 p.m. The soft drinks and a few uneaten treats were cleared away. Nobody lingered. Tomorrow was another day of training.

Vanishing from Lake Issyk-Kul before dawn was never going to be easy. When they had talked the plan through back in Moscow and on the phone with Seppelt, it had all seemed feasible. But now everything felt terrifying. Yuliya felt the tension in her head and her stomach. Vitaly's quiet determination almost undid her. It would just take one person to put two and two together. All those little jokes about whether or not Yuliya was taping people? What if those jests were held up to the light in the morning? And now you are telling me that they have just vanished?

They went back to their room and began packing their bags. The last time they had packed was in the short stopover in Moscow when they had returned to their apartment in the middle of the night between flights. It seemed an age since they had spent any time in their own home among their own things. They would never be doing that again.

Vitaly took care of entertaining Robert as Yuliya crammed everything into bags solemnly. When they left the room with these bags, tiptoeing out into the darkness, they would be drawing a line under their lives as they had lived them until now. There would be no going back. Their excuses would buy a few days in Moscow to tidy up, but they were all in. When they walked out of this hotel they wouldn't tiptoe into the darkness, they would leap into the unknown. If Vitaly was worried by the prospect, he wasn't showing it, so Yuliya kept her thoughts to herself.

Sleep was shallow and fleeting. They went to bed at 2 a.m. with the alarm set for a little before 5 a.m. A few days earlier, while Yuliya and the crew were training, Vitaly had wandered off the hotel grounds in search of a suitable taxi driver. He had made an arrangement with a man who drove a roomy estate car and was willing to show up at their hotel well before dawn.

From their first-floor room, Vitaly and Yuliya could see the moonlit lake and, if the sky was clear, the dark shapes of the mountains on the far shore. They could also see the main gate of the hotel. Cars were not allowed through, so in the darkness they just sat and waited and watched. When Vitaly had arranged for them to meet the taxi at the front gate, he had imagined that discretion was built into the arrangement. At 5 a.m. in the dark, what could go wrong? Now, though, the street lights seemed treacherously bright and the front of the hotel itself was too well-lit.

Uniformed security guards patrolled like roaming wolves. Any excitement would attract them. Kazarin was billeted two floors above them, sharing exactly the same view of the road and lake. The room on the floor in between was occupied by another athlete. If one person noticed the Stepanovs stealing towards the roadway with their belongings and their infant son in the middle of the night, who knew what unpleasantness would follow.

They made their way downstairs earlier than they had planned, as Vitaly feared the estate car arriving and blasting its horn to alert them of its presence. It was still dark but not nearly dark enough. And it was a struggle to drag the big bags, to pull the pram and to carry Robert. Robert needed to be kept calm and happy. His first squall of distress would be like a factory siren. They passed through the deserted lobby and out into the cold air, still trying not to drag the bags or the pram, still tip-toeing with Robert, still whispering to each other. Inevitably, their leaving caught the attention of a security guard.

'Have you paid for your room?'

They didn't have any papers at all relating to their stay. Kazarin had said that everything would be fixed up at the end of the camp, the part that the Federation was paying and the extra charge covering Vitaly and Robert's stay. The nature of their departure being what it was, they hadn't been in a position to go to Kazarin and tell him that they wanted to fix everything up now. In the darkness there was no option but to front it out.

'Of course we have paid.'

'Well, let me check and call reception.'

'Go ahead.'

The security men jabbed a number into his phone. At that moment the taxi pulled up outside the main gate. The driver had his formidable turret of a wife installed in the passenger seat, riding shotgun for the long journey. It was not a time for being choosy about company. Vitaly and Yuliya just wanted to get in the car.

There had been nobody at reception when Yuliya and Vitaly had tiptoed past. And now there was nobody answering the phone. A blessed relief. They kept moving towards the gate as the phone kept ringing. The voices, the sound of the car, doors opening . . . surely somebody was going to wake up and take a look outside.

'Keep walking,' Vitaly hissed to Yuliya. 'Whatever happens with reception happens. Keep walking and we just get in the car.'

With his phone still to his ear, the security guard began walking towards the hotel to check out the situation for himself. The taxi driver had the back of the estate car open and ready to receive everything that was hurled into it from the darkness. He had the impression now that this was no ordinary departure. On the other hand, it was none of his business as long as he got paid. As the last door shut, the vehicle was already pulling away. Nobody looked back to see if there was a security man chasing them down the road with an invoice.

The drive was long and uncomfortable. With the driver's wife lodged sourly in the front passenger seat, Yuliya and Vitaly were cramped in the back, separated by Robert in his car seat. There were some stretches of good road between Lake Issyk-Kul and Bishkek. There was a lot of bad road too, surfaces pocked with potholes that they bounced in and out of with a violence seemingly undiminished by any shock absorbers. Dawn had broken and in silence they gazed out at this strange country they would never see again.

It was 150 miles to Bishkek and Manas airport. It took five hours, and the Kazarin group were already waking up to the news that the people they had thrown a party for the previous evening had vanished into thin air. Yuliya's phone was buzzing with calls and texts from Kazarin long before they reached the airport. After a while, the least stressful course was just to switch the phone off.

They had another five hours to wait for their flight. Robert was struggling with a fever, and Yuliya and Vitaly were dog-tired. Five more hours. Divorce would have been easier. They settled into a couple of seats in the departure area. A young couple with a baby, five hours early for a flight. What was their story? Thankfully, nobody asked them that, but they asked each other.

Chapter 32

For five hours they weren't sure what to be afraid of, so they were a little bit afraid of everything. Loitering passengers. Fussing airport workers. Women who stopped to admire Robert.

Who knew how their disappearance was being digested back at the hotel? What alarms bells were sounding in paranoid brains? What calls had been made? It was either just another episode in the tiresome soap opera of Yuliya from Kursk and her nuisance husband. Or it was an emergency.

Robert slept a little and they envied him. They were jangling with excitement and nerves, and sleep would have to ambush them later.

'Why did you stick with me?' Yuliya asked suddenly.

He was used to her directness but it was seldom so introspective. Usually it was more like 'Why are you such an idiot, Vitaly?'

'That's not the question,' he said. She had always been the white feather that he was going to scoop up and keep. 'I saw you from the start. All you are. The question is: why did you marry me? Why did you even keep seeing me?'

She looked around the terminal and, although it had come to life a couple of hours ago, her concentration seemed to still the busyness of it. She had his full attention.

'Do you remember the morning when you drove me to the airport?'

'That?'

'No. That was just a taxi fare you saved me.'

She pauses again. Then she tells him about the day that fol-lowed. Three flights. Fifteen hours of travelling. Just to get to Castres in France. It was dark when she got to her room and it struck her that she had nobody to call. Nobody to tell her day to. When she got up the next morning it was sunny. She was far from home in a country she didn't know and she was all alone.

'Was that the life I wanted?'

She had decided that she had to start getting things in order. First job: ditch her agent. Sergey would have to walk the plank. That would be the start of the new Yuliya.

She had wanted a successful career. It wasn't easy. In the beginning there had been the curse of shin splints. Then, when the shin splints went away, tuberculosis arrived. TB and all those dreary months in hospital. She got better but when she'd gone back to training it wasn't the same. She felt feverish all the time. Weak as a kitten. She had lost her old strength. The doctors insisted that her lungs were fine. If it wasn't her lungs, well, then what was it? Was it in her head? She was scared.

Vitaly checked on Robert and turned back to listen some more, fearing he had heard this story before and hadn't much liked it. She'd been in hospital . . . Mokhnev had come to see her . . . She'd liked that . . . She was weak . . . And that was how she'd started taking drugs. Life had just happened to her.

But now she veered left.

'You know Katia's mother-in-law, yes? Nina?'

He knew Nina more by reputation, but he was listening. He nodded.

'Well, she's a devout Christian. She believes it all, but she's okay. I respect her. Anyway, Katia had told her that I was still weak and she told Katia that she knew somebody who could fix me. She knew this woman who could cure anything.'

Aha. This was something else that he loved about Yuliya. She had faith in the exact science of chemistry to the extent that she would permit her body to be trespassed upon by pills and pointy needles. Simultaneously she could believe in the powers of an old crone who claimed to be able to cure anything. This old crone lived about an hour's drive west of Kursk, in a town called Kurchatov, and at the first opportunity Yuliya took the bus journey to see her.

'I was the first to arrive. I was two hours early. Nobody in the waiting room. I had to sit there for about two and a half hours while other people went in and out. I was looking at them as they left her, just to see if they looked fixed or happy. Eventually it was my turn. All I could see when I went in was these shelves with religious icons on them looking down at me. And then this woman started asking questions.

'"What is the problem with you?"

"I feel sick all the time," I told her.

"I can see one of your lungs. It is in a fog. Something is not right."

"But maybe there is something else causing the fever," I said. I couldn't believe that. She knew my lungs weren't right. She could see a fog.'

I bet she could, thought Vitaly, *and a sucker walking through the fog*. Instead, he asked what Yuliya had wanted the old crone to say.

'To be honest, I wanted her to say that I would run in the next Olympics and that I would do well.'

'And?'

'She didn't. She told me not to waste my time going looking for another woman like her. She knew what was going to happen in my life. She could see a picture of me, and in the picture I was married and she said the man I was with was giving me his hand. She said the first time he offers me his hand

I don't take it. But she sees me happy and laughing and I have two kids with this man.'

'So that was it. She told a young woman that she would get married? Were you happy about that?'

'No, I asked her straight if I would have success as a runner.'

'And?'

'She said, "Why are you running? You don't need running. Have a husband. Have kids." And I said no, I was a professional. That it was my job being a runner. I had to run. And she shook her head and she told me that I would have some success if I run, but not much. She saw me lying down, upset by many injuries, not happy with running.'

'Not what you wanted to hear?'

'Exactly. So that was why I believed her.'

'Oh.'

'If she was a fake she would tell me what I wanted to hear. But she didn't. And she didn't know that deep down I didn't have full faith in my career then either. She couldn't know that. So that was good what she told me. And after that I started looking out for the man she had told me about.'

Vitaly looked at the woman he had married. How strange it was to be absorbing this as they sat about fidgeting on a five-hour delay in their escape from their old life. Would he ever stop learning new things about her?

'So then,' Yuliya continued, 'about two months later I thought, "Yes, I have found the man."'

'And that was me.'

'No,' she said, 'it wasn't.'

She told him about getting off a bus one day close to where she trained in Kursk and how, as she had alighted, a man had approached her in his car and called to her through his rolled-down window. He introduced himself as Andrey. His car identified him as a taxi driver. He said that he'd seen her getting on the bus so many stops before and he had instantly fallen for her. Head over heels. He had been tracking the bus, stopping at every stop, driving on in hope until eventually he had seen her get off.

Vitaly scrunched up his face.

'So you ran? Called the cops?'

'No,' she said. 'I got in.'

She said she thought that this stalking taxi driver had to be the very man predicted to come into her life by the all-healing lady of Kurchatov. Wasn't the pursuit of the bus his courtly way of stretching out his hand? So they had dated four or five times and Yuliya got to know Andrey better, but he had not been so courtly and not at all who she thought he might be. He would not be her husband nor the father of her two children. At the time, she simply believed she must have misread things through eagerness. It could not be the case that the visionary lady of Kurchatov had faulty reception.

It was July 2009 when the meter stopped running with the taxi driver. The following month she had met Vitaly, and a couple of weeks after that they had dated for the first time. And then, in pensive mood at a window in her hotel room in Castres, she had fallen to wondering if he could be the one, the future husband. Their first date had been spent mostly in the car but he had been kind and attentive.

'You see, you opened the car door for me. That was the kind of man the Kurchatov lady talked about. You were kind. You listened to me. Men always confuse waiting for their turn to talk again with listening. You didn't. You listened.'

'I never knew all that,' he said. 'I thought that you just thought that I was an idiot.'

Her face was sideways to him as she checked on Robert, and he wondered for a second if she was about to cry. *Don't push your luck, Vitaly. She's not that girl.* She looked at him now, and in her gaze he saw what he used to see before her injury, when he was her rabbit and she was running him into the ground every day. Determination. Pure.

'I did think that. But you were a nice idiot. And you saved me a taxi fare.'

On that Tuesday morning in Castres, she had known she was going to see him again. And that she was looking forward to it.

For the first time, here at Manas airport of all places, Vitaly fully understood the history of their relationship. He'd always had a chance and he always would.

~

In Sheremetyevo airport they took the escalator down from the second floor of the arrivals hall and sleepwalked through passport control. They had officially entered their own country again. For the last time. Nobody paid them any attention. Another escalator down to the luggage hall. Vitaly pushed Robert in his pram and they wandered to the conveyor belt, while Yuliya found a quiet spot under the angle of the escalator and called Kazarin. They talked for five minutes. She came back to Vitaly and her eyes were watery.

Kazarin had been hostile.

'I don't need these kind of athletes,' he told her. 'I am here to train you, not to deal with your personal life. It is about the work you are doing. You cannot just do that. You cannot just walk away.'

She had explained that the problem was Vitaly. Had everybody not seen how he had been at the party for his own son? He was unhappy. She was going to have to sort things out.

'I am going to deal with my husband soon and I will be back in a few days.'

On reflection, the conversation hadn't gone any worse than she would have expected, but the gathering tension of all the sleepless hours had drained her. They collected their luggage, soothed Robert and walked to the train. They were so weary that it took Vitaly a moment or two to work out which day it was. They would be departing Russia on 23 November, so . . .

'We've got three days left in Russia. Do we sit around or do we want to try and record some more people?'

She looked at him in disbelief. She had just lost her career, her baby was sick, she had spent the last ten days surreptitiously taping teammates and coaches, they had fled in the night and remained awake for twenty-four hours, they had been cold half the time, frightened all the time. In three days they would be fleeing their own country. They had yet to pack or make arrangements beyond their air tickets. They hadn't even reached their own apartment and drawn breath. And all he wanted to talk about right now was more taping.

'Yuliya, look,' he said. 'Okay, the coach of the Olympic champion is giving out steroids . . . It is good but it's not enough. We have still got to have an Olympic champion talking as well. We need to talk to Mariya and tape her.'

Yuliya was angry now. When he said 'we', of course, he meant her. This was too much, though. Savinova had been kind and gracious to Yuliya. Recently it seemed their friendship had grown. She had admired Savinova and she had measured herself against her. It had been such a relief that Mariya hadn't been at Lake Issyk-Kul and the training camp. Maybe this horrible task would never get done.

'You just do whatever you want,' she replied.

He could see she was angry with him but, without Russia's Olympic golden girl, the entire exercise might pass unnoticed. Savinova would be the tipping point for WADA. Yes, Mariya was lovely but principle was principle, Vitaly argued. Just because Savinova was an essentially decent and nice person, it didn't give them the right to spare her and let down all the other essentially decent and nice athletes who raced clean and finished behind her. It would have to be done.

'How?' Yuliya said. 'I've never been to Mariya's apartment.'

Gently, he took Yuliya's phone from her hands and began texting while she tended to Robert. She looked up after a while. He was still texting.

'Who are you texting?'

'Savinova.'

'Savinova?'

'Yeah. I've chatted with her a few times before online. But now I'm just texting her.'

'Why? What are you telling her?'

'I'm not telling her anything. You are. You are telling her that you have a problem, that you need to speak with her.'

'Oh Vitaly. Shit. Fuck you. I don't want to do that.'

'It is arranged.'

They finished the long journey in silence.

～

She took the train the next day from Kazansky station. They had done some packing that morning. Packing and the antici-pation of being on the way to somewhere new used to be fun for Yuliya. This time there was nothing enjoyable. There was a clock ticking and they were short on time for everything. This was escape without escapism. She just knew to pack the most important things and leave the rest. They would be leaving for a long time. They had barely slept and their body clocks were haywire. She felt like a zombie walking through her own life.

The train was a fifty-minute journey to Podolsk, the indus-trial town where Savinova had an apartment. Yuliya fretted all the way. This wasn't just scary, it was also unpleasant. Her heart hoped that her phone would fail to record or that Savinova would clam up. Her head knew that Vitaly was right.

They had argued. He agreed that Savinova was a good person. A friend. But he kept saying Mariya had had a choice back at the beginning. Yuliya knew in her heart that, for the Yuliyas and Mariyas, that choice was never as clear as Vitaly was making out. Down the road, Vitaly said, Savinova would still have a choice. She was an Olympic champion. Lots of good people had finished behind her in lots of races. She could just come out and tell her story.

And would Yuliya have any credibility if it emerged that she had spared her friends? Wasn't that the root of the problem? Wasn't that what Russia did? Protect the champions while offering up some sacrificial lambs? Giving Savinova a pass while Bazdyreva got recorded. Savinova was a good person but she had made a choice. Yuliya should know that. She lived in a country where connections were better than currency. How often had they talked about that? Yuliya couldn't put the big fish back in the water just because it was a very friendly fish. This would have to be done.

Still, Yuliya thought, *still*. She saw herself as the scrappy little outsider from Kursk who had brought the baggage of her husband to camps. A lot of people hated her. A lot of them had never given her a chance, but Savinova was different. Kind. Open. She'd taken Yuliya in. For some reason, she'd wanted Yuliya to succeed. They had walked and talked, two women discussing babies and relationships and life. And now she had to do this to her?

Mariya answered the door, hugged Yuliya and beckoned her in.

Kazarin had called her from Lake Issyk-Kul and told her that Yuliya had gone. Disappeared. He had got up and she just wasn't there any more. Yuliya repeated the story that Vitaly had starting spinning by text the previous day. That they had been fighting about the pills. That Vitaly had said Yuliya would never learn. Kazarin was giving her more pills before she had even finished her ban. The next sanction would be for life. Was that what she wanted to tell their son? He was talking about moving them all to America. Maybe she could run clean over there.

Savinova leaned forward sympathetically.

'You have to separate your work and your personal life,' she told Yuliya, 'for your own sake.'

'Uh huh.'

'Private life should never affect your work. Otherwise, you will never achieve anything.'

Yuliya went on. At camp she was slower than everybody else. She needed to get back to being the old Yuliya. She needed to make money, to race again, to travel to big championships. Was there any choice? She owed it to her son to take the pills. Savinova shook her head. There was just no other way. And so she began telling Yuliya the facts of a running life.

'There is no other way to do it. Everyone in Russia is on pharma.'

She herself knew that it was bad for her health, she said, but no one that she had seen had ever had any real problems. Yuliya had been listening to this argument right from the beginning. Mokhnev used to tell her about the steroids he took back in the old Soviet days when he was steeplechasing. Never did him any harm, he always said. *Except that your brain is made of straw*, she would think to herself.

'The dosage levels aren't that of horses,' Savinova said.

Maybe the solution was simple. Be smarter. Yuliya asked her about wash-out periods. Savinova said she had learned that, when the coaches gave you the number of days for drugs like Oral Turinabol, oxandrolone or Parabolan to clear the system, they were talking about the worst-case scenario. And the worst-case scenario was for the throwers, those big old whales with their slow metabolisms and fat arses. If you were small and skinny and running and sweating hard every day, like her or Yuliya, the stuff vanished a lot quicker. When recounting the details, often Savinova would refer to her husband Alexey's guidance and advice. Her faith in Lekha, as she called him now, was always touching.

Yuliya brought up the topic of human growth hormone. They had spoken about it in Kislovodsk.

'Well,' she said to Savinova, 'you trained on the hormone.'

'I did it but, you see, Lekha advised me, because he was drying me out. Yes, he did a good job drying me out.'

The chat about drugs and life within the system came easily, but Savinova was mindful of the bigger picture. She was heart-breakingly empathetic. What about solving Yuliya and Vitaly's troubles? And smoothing things with Kazarin? There were ways of making everybody happy here, she thought.

'You have to talk. You have to try, using all the truths and untruths you can muster . . .'

That made sense, but the bottom line was unchanged. As Savinova had said, there was no other way but pharma. And for Vitaly there was no other way but clean.

'Tell me what I can do, Mariya.'

It was time to consult on a broader basis. Savinova had an endearing habit of giving pet names to the people in her life that she liked. She summoned Alexey, who had briefly come into the room earlier but then had wandered off.

'Lyosh, we have a question. In short, Yulka has got problems, in that Vitalik is against pharma. Totally against it.'

Yulka and Vitalik. The sheer affection of it made Yuliya want to cry.

Alexey was no relationship counsellor. He joined the chat but the question that had drawn him in was lost. Their conversation returned to its own natural rhythms, the things athletes speak about when relaxed and among their peers. Well, Russian athletes.

Yuliya played the role that suited her circumstance. The kid who didn't know too much. She had questions. They had answers. Why? What? How? When? Really? She would ask the questions. Sometimes Savinova would answer. More often they would turn their faces expectantly towards Alexey, who was like their search engine for all matters doping.

TB500? Is that detectable? Not yet but they are trying to develop the test. You tan more easily with it. Did you see Irina? She took a course of TB and we saw her on a start line and people thought that she was a black girl.

Americans? They reach a very high level on their own health, and then they start to add. But that is how it should be, really.

Kenyans? When the testers come I've heard that they just run into the mountains. I heard that too.

WADA? Athletes, generally, are sick people. I mean, if WADA is shut down, then people will actually be dying, for real ... Yes, that will happen. People will die.

Alcohol? The latest aid to doping in Russia. It facilitates faster absorption. It drives it out of the body ... You don't swallow, you just have it in your mouth. You walk about a bit, and rinse your mouth ... And that is it, you spit it out? Yes.[1]

Micro-dosing? Minimal doses, 500 or 300 a day if you choose micro-doses. Maybe more to get up to speed.

Alexey was an encyclopaedia about doping and the world beyond their own borders. He had the technical fluency of an academic, an expertise that surpassed the limits of a Portugalov or a Kazarin.

'The stimulation index is calculated specifically from the reticulocytes. The reticulocytes are not specifically matured erythrocytes. That is, you put them in, and you get, for example ... That is, you did not use them, and you had a certain level of those reticulocytes ... You use it, and they immediately matured very quickly, and then, right off, you got it, there was an increase. And that is the level you usually have. So straight away, just like that … That is, it is immediately visible. If they take some from you, your reticulocytes are above a certain level, because the body is programmed to have reticulocytes of average fluorescence, that is, they sort of matured in the middle of the high fluorescence, when they already mature, they convert into erythrocytes, and low fluorescence, when they are only barely in embryonic form.'

Oh yeah, thought Yuliya, *that's just what I thought*.

Alexey recalled the winter when Savinova had been doing hormones and things had gotten very tough. The testers had been calling several times a month, he said. Very rough. Savinova added that the testers were still calling. She knew she'd be having two more tests before the New Year.

Yuliya looked at the two of them. *They are like a differently mutated version of myself and Vitaly*, she thought. When Yuliya had been paying her money to Portugalov, she had taken the chance on him being her only source of information. Savinova had paid Portugalov but had always been primarily guided by her husband and his concern for her career and her well-being.

They just had to work with Portugalov, Savinova said, use him. You needed to make sure you were covered with the tests and that there were no surprises. You paid these people money and pretended you were doing what they were saying to do, but actually you might be doing something else. In the end it was she and her husband deciding how she would dope. You just made sure that they covered your back but always remembered that you were the one running, the one risking your health, your reputation and your career.

'Dope smart' was Alexey's mantra. 'Don't dope at all' was Vitaly's mantra.

It was sweet to look at these two and see something of herself and Vitaly in them.

Every Russian girl grew up with the fairy tale of Ruslan and Ludmila, the story of the brave knight questing in search of the princess abducted by an evil wizard. In Pushkin's poem the narrator said that the tale was told to him by a learned cat. Every girl was entranced by the notion of her own Ruslan. In their own ways, she and Mariya had found theirs.

When Yuliya left Savinova's apartment it was past 7 p.m. This woman was so open. So friendly. Of all the runners who had been cold with her, jealous of her or dismissive of her because of who she married or where she had come from, Savinova was the one who looked past all that and just wanted good things for her. To Savinova there was no Yuliya and Vitaly. There was Yulka and Vitalik. It made Yuliya smile again just to think of that.

Walking towards the train station, she struggled to keep herself together. She called Vitaly and told him. This was too much. Too far.

'Was it a good recording?' he asked.

Yes. It was a good recording, yes, good evidence. And yes, he would like it.

'But please, Vitaly, is there a way that we don't ever use this recording? Please.'

'Look,' he said, 'come home and we will talk.'

It was 19 November. Tick . . . tick . . . tick . . . She knew there would be no time for talking.

Sobbing, she waited for her train to come. On the train she sat and brooded, hating what she had just done. What was killing her was what she had got on her phone. It was good material and that was why she felt so bad.

She wanted to delete it.

But she couldn't.

Chapter 33

Usually little Robert was sunshine in a pram but these past few days he hadn't been himself and Yuliya was worried. Vitaly had loose ends he needed to tie up. Everything was happening too quickly. She was surprised when Vitaly came to her and said he thought they should try to tape Portugalov before they left. She hadn't seen Portugalov in the longest time. Their parting had been unpleasant. Portugalov pretending pathetically that he had moved to another job. Idiot.

And she was tired. So tired. Physically, emotionally, spiritually. She'd lost count of the number of people she had trapped. These last few weeks she seesawed from whistle-blower to informer. The anxiety. The lies. Robert. Savinova. Things were fraying her nerves. And now one more tape? Were they going to push this until they got caught? The consequences didn't bear thinking about.

'How would we tape Portugalov? When? How? Why? It's stupid.'

'Today. You just call on him. Just imagine if you could get him to start boasting about all the medallists he has created. All of them. Those stars in all those sports? Proof that it's much more than athletics.'

'To me? He's going to boast to me? Vitaly, he hates you and he doesn't much like me. Robert isn't well. We have only half packed. There is no reason for me to call on Portugalov. This is mad. Just no.'

It was a twenty-minute walk from the apartment to the VNIIFK Institute, the All Russian Research Institute of Physical Culture and Sport, near Kursky station. They went while it was still morning, swaddling themselves and Robert against the mean Moscow winter. As they walked, Vitaly was on the phone to Seppelt, negotiating a little breathing space. Just one more day in Moscow? To pack, to tie things up. Okay.

They were wrapped up so thoroughly that members of their own family wouldn't have recognised them but, given Portugalov's paranoia, it was wise to keep Vitaly out of sight altogether. There was a small grocery store in the basement of a nearby building on the same side of the street. Vitaly would hang back there with Robert, stealing the warmth as he pretended to browse the potatoes and cabbages. From there, he could keep half an eye on the building. Just in case.

'Just in case what, Vitaly?'

'I don't know. Just in case. This is Moscow.'

The VNIIFK ('Devoted to the Service of Russian Sports Science') was a squat building, an architectural souvenir of the Soviet seventies. Security was one guy at a desk like a bored old *dezhurnaya* back in the day. Her phone already recording, Yuliya announced that she was popping in to see Dr Portugalov.

'He's there. Third floor,' the guard said without glancing up.

Portugalov was busy and not pleased to see Yuliya. No outstretched arms. No outstretched hand.

'Well, what have you got to say?'

'How are things with you?'

'Tell me how things are with *you*. Otherwise I'll be under the impression that you've only come to see me after two years to find out how things are with me. Well?'

'Well, I had a baby.'

'Now that's an event.'

She had agreed with Vitaly that she should refer to her

husband merely as an unfortunate part of her life that she was willing to purge if necessary. Otherwise, she should keep it simple. She would remind Portugalov that not too long ago he had told her she was faster than Savinova, that she could run 1:55. Well, she was back now, and she wanted to run fast. Would he work with her? If he demurred, she would add that she now recognised Vitaly was a pain in the arse. If Portugalov asked, she would say that she was happy to divorce Vitaly in a heartbeat. To get to Rio? Anything. Surely that would be a sonata to Portugalov's old ears.

He was curt. He conveyed his distaste for her and the casual impertinence of this drop-in. What had she been doing since the baby had been born? Not baby news, please. What had she been doing about her running?

What did she need to do, she asked?

'Speed and strength work, if you've started, only just started. Well, it's still early. And are you taking part in the trials?'

'Yes.'

'And the baby?'

'Is with me.'

'Is it going with you?'

'Well, my husband is acting as nanny.'

'Rotten, huh?'

'Well, my husband is being nanny.'

'So the child will be getting a rotten childhood, always travelling to training camps and races and never being home.'

Portugalov's animosity to Vitaly was still fresh and vivid.

She said she would be returning to Lake Issyk-Kul the next day. Her baby had been sick. She'd had to come home but she was heading back for the last two weeks of camp. Portugalov flinched at her stupidity. It took days to acclimatise. What was the point? She felt like an idiot. Had she raised some flags in his brain?

He said that if it was what she wanted she should come back to the Institute when she returned to Moscow. She could do tests to establish where her fitness was at. He wasn't saying he would take her back under his wing, just that the facilities would be available. She should bring a sample along also. Those sort of tests would also be part of the day. She would need to stay in Moscow for a bit, maybe test herself on the second day after the mountains.

'Hi, Alexei. Or on the second day.'

Yuliya jumped. Alexei Melnikov had just walked into the office behind her. Why were these people always strolling into each other's offices unannounced? What the fuck was he doing here? His office was miles away. Had he spoken with Kazarin?

'Hi!' said Melnikov.

'Hi,' said Yuliya as if this was an unexpected delight.

'After the mountains—' continued Portugalov.

'Why did you leave the trials so early?' Melnikov interrupted. He still loved to dominate conversations. He had no concern for others' boredom. His arrival gave Portugalov the excuse he needed to clam up. Yuliya sat and listened in despondency. More Melnikov on tape was something they didn't need. They had enough for a greatest hits compilation.

'My baby fell ill,' she muttered. 'Some sort of poisoning. A high temperature.'

'I told you the child would have a poisoned childhood,' Portugalov said sourly.

Melnikov talked on. He told Yuliya that this year in the winter season she was not to dope. Just prepare without dope. She thought about Kazarin and his fistful of blue bullets intended as her starter course for the season. That disclosure would only blow the conversation further off course. Over her head Portugalov enquired of Melnikov if the 'bad things' were over for Yuliya. On 28 January they will be, Yuliya said, engaging directly with Portugalov again.

'I just don't know if we should do anything this winter,' said

Melnikov, jumping in again. 'She has reinstatement doping controls.'

Portugalov wasn't convinced. On they went, two old fools bluffing each other. She wasn't to worry. He, Melnikov, and his good friend Portugalov, being serious and intelligent men, would be getting to the bottom of this whole blood passport business. He wanted to make clear that he was still the man. He was still arranging doping controls when Rusada came or when IDTM were sniffing around. The advance notice service was still in operation.

Yuliya watched them like a witness to a duel. She said she had concerns about how much Kazarin knew.

'I also talked about this with Masha [Savinova]. She says that he doesn't particularly know anything.'

Melnikov was like a hungry trout spotting a fat hooked worm. 'About what?'

'About, well . . . The pharmacological side of the preparations.'

Melnikov exploded into a scoffing fit.

'Come off it, he doesn't know! He's got his own preparations. I talked with him in detail. I'll talk with him in detail. About you. It's just that now it's not the time.'

Portugalov listened sourly, really not interested in talk about Yuliya.

Yuliya addressed him directly.

'There's also another question that's worried me since my last conversation with you. The fact that these steroid passports have now appeared.'

Again Melnikov jumped in.

'They're not in force yet. But they're coming into force. The Russian Anti-Doping Agency in particular is sniffing around, collecting data.'

'Well, that's a different conversation, Alexei,' said Portugalov, shifting uncomfortably.

'That's not for now,' Melnikov nodded. 'That's for later. For now, it doesn't affect you.'

Had Portugalov smelled a rat? Was he clamming up, letting Melnikov hang himself like a fool? Not for the first time, she felt the tension of deceit be soothed by the sedative tone of Melnikov's voice. Melnikov wanted her to know that it was business as usual. That the business with all the bans was behind everybody now.

'If we were not caught blind on this thing [the ABP blood passport] . . . Yuliya, try to understand us . . . If they would have told us at least 10 per cent how it would be done, we would never . . . Besides . . .'

Portugalov's broody silence was stifling the conversation. Yuliya asked directly if it would be possible to be prepared by Portugalov again. Yet again Melnikov answered. Of course. When they had the possibilities of the additional doping testing to check everything, even blood, maybe then . . .

By now Melnikov was the only person interested in conversation. Yuliya's plan had fallen apart once Melnikov had entered the room and now he wouldn't shut up. Finally, Portugalov asked Melnikov irritably if he had finished with 'the girl'. He had. It was time to get rid of her.

'I hope we'll be able to work together,' said Yuliya brightly to both men as she backed out of the office.

'I hope so, I hope so,' said Melnikov. 'As they say, youth is fed by hope.'

Portugalov, not saying a word, seemed nauseous.

That was a lot of risk for not very much, thought Yuliya. *Thanks, Melnikov.*

~

Fleeing Russia now, they flew to Prague before dawn. Their homeland down below them held all their history, their previous lives, their families, their friends, their personal moments. All down there on the vanishing vastness. From Prague they would be moving on immediately. Would they ever know a sense of home again?

They had left the apartment at 3 a.m. Quietly lest they woke Igor and Olga. Vitaly knew that his brother must have guessed something. All those calls in English to Seppelt? Igor must have eavesdropped. Family was like KGB but more in your face. If it meant having the apartment to themselves, he imagined that Igor didn't care very much what Vitaly was plotting. Vitaly blanked it all from his mind, though. There was still work to do.

Yuliya could better live in the moment. She wondered if they would ever return to Russia. If she was leaving a part of herself behind. They had packed light apart from Robert's warehouse of necessities.

'Two bags each,' Vitaly teased. 'Mine took three hours to pack. Yours took fifteen hours.'

Maybe that was all they would need. Maybe she was over-thinking things. A documentary in Germany? Some people would hear about it, of course they would, but Yuliya reckoned the fuss would soon die down. People had lives filled with other worries. In a year or two, less even, they might be at the summer races in a Moscow park with friends. They would be laughing about the entire mad thing and nobody would know or care who they were. Then she thought about the people she'd secretly recorded, their anger, their influence. That summer evening at a Moscow park just disappeared.

There would be training opportunities in Germany or America or wherever they found themselves. Though she had no idea what the point of training might be. She might never see Russia again, let alone race in the nation's colours.

She dandled Robert on her lap. Kissed the top of his fair head. Would he even speak Russian, this little American fellow?

Life was so simple for him. If he wanted to cry, he cried. If he wanted to eat, he ate. If he wanted to be changed, he cried again. He could have all the attention he wanted. Every moment with him was good and every moment was distracting. She would focus on what she had, not on what she was leaving behind. Everything was going to be all right.

The flight to Prague took three hours. They took a taxi from the airport to the main railway station, catching glimpses of the city they had read about. Where was Wenceslas Square? The Charles Bridge? The postcard stuff? The station was old and the area looked as if the Great Patriotic War had just ended. The taxi driver wanted fifty euros. In some ways all cities were the same. People everywhere on the make. Fifty euros for 10 kilometres? Vitaly asked for a receipt and kept it for Seppelt.

After another train journey of five and a half hours, they pulled in to Berlin's gleaming train station. They took another taxi and called Seppelt.

'We are in a taxi now and on the way to your studio.'

Seppelt was out on the pavement when they arrived. He was busy. Here were the keys to his apartment. He was staying with his mother again. He would see Vitaly back here bright and early in the morning. The taxi drove on.

Chapter 34

They would be in Germany for ten days before the documentary aired. Vitaly worked away on the transcriptions. There was one late debate about whether athletes would be included in the documentary at all. Weren't they all victims, Seppelt's boss suggested?

'We are talking about systematic doping here,' Vitaly said, 'and so are the athletes victims or are they part of it? In the end, I believe they are part of it. They are not victims.'

They moved on.

It felt as though there was no longer a clock ticking. Now it was a burning fuse. The documentary went to air on 3 December 2014. ARD were required by law to notify everybody who would be implicated in the film. Most of the notifications went out by email. For some reason, on the day the emails went out, Vitaly and Yuliya had taken each other's phones. Vitaly noticed he had Yuliya's phone when Savinova's number started appearing. Then a series of unknown numbers.

He was advised to remove the SIM card from the phone before his location could be identified. He called Yuliya and told her to do the same. They pulled the SIM cards, switched the phones off and abandoned them until early in the New Year. By Wednesday 3 December the network had been trailing ads for the documentary for days. Online in the Russian media Yuliya and Vitaly were already pariahs.

Vitaly called Yuliya.

'Hey, look, you are famous already and it hasn't even aired.'

She spoke no German so she wouldn't be following the film closely when it aired. Hopefully Robert would distract her as he needed to be looked after. She was happy to just wait for events to unravel in their own time.

Christoph Kopp, the Berlin sports administrator who had made introductions for them in the past, was with them. He had called in the afternoon on another pretext but he stayed to watch the documentary. Typical of the many kindnesses he had already done them.

Vitaly had seen most of the film already, so he designated himself chief babysitter and looked after Robert while Yuliya watched with Christoph. Kopp didn't speak Russian, whereas Yuliya's English was poor and her German non-existent. It was odd for everybody. She looked away when she saw Savinova's face. She had asked Seppelt and had begged Vitaly to please leave Mariya out. But Savinova was their big fish. If only Yuliya had done better with Portugalov. Maybe she could have spared Mariya.

From what she could gather, overall Seppelt had done a fine job. But it was impossible to know what to feel. They were a slingshot, and the small rock they had launched might sail through the air with a whistle heard only by them. Or it might hit the giant between the eyes and all hell would break loose before he hit the ground. Or this broadcast in German could be a small anecdote they would tell their grandchildren someday. 'That's Grandma when she was young and we were on the television.' Or it could be the border between the first half of their lives and what remained. Deep down, they knew they had crossed a line and there was no going back. Nothing in the future would ever be the same as the things in their past. RUSADA, WADA, IAAF, IOC, all the letters of the alphabet, all the organisations and institutions. Vitaly, Yuliya and Robert were just husband, wife and child practically alone in a big and dangerous world.

When Yuliya checked social media later on she wished that she hadn't. The online word was black with hatred for her. She was a villain, a whore, a traitor and a coward, a death waiting to occur. This was a far more powerful reaction than she had ever imagined, but she knew in her heart how Russia worked. The emptiest vessels made the most tweets. It was in silence, when you were relaxed and unguarded, that the real trouble came.

People were tweeting that if Yuliya Stepanova ever came back to Russia they would kill her. Fine. It was the ones they would send *from* Russia to kill her that she worried about. From polonium to poisoned umbrella tips, assassination was a Russian art form she didn't want to consider. Every time she checked her computer, the hatred was more intense. People stoking each other's spite. In the days that followed, Vitaly went on the internet more than she did. He followed the Russian political reaction closely but he showed her their names and their faces on the front pages around the world. Little details about their lives were beginning to seep out.

She just wanted to sleep until she had been forgotten.

What had they done? Herself and the nerdy guy from the Outreach desk?

The Strange Story of Ekaterina Antilskaya – Part Two

During their last days in Moscow, Antilskaya's name was on Vitaly and Yuliya's to-do list.

It had bothered them that the woman who managed IDTM's operation in Russia was still in a job. Two and a half years before, when WADA had wanted Yuliya tested, they'd authorised

IDTM to collect the blood and urine samples. Antilskaya was IDTM's woman in Moscow. What happened next demonstrated the sham of elite drug testing in Russia.

If Yuliya had run rings around Antilskaya back then, it hadn't been difficult. Antilskaya had been happily complicit. She had misrepresented the time and location of the test and claimed expenses that hadn't been incurred. She hadn't bothered to watch Yuliya deliver her sample. The only rule was that the rules didn't matter. Vitaly had passed all this on to WADA, who had paid a lot of money to get the test done.

Nothing had changed. Ekaterina Antilskaya was still doing business as usual. Now, two and a half years later, Yuliya's ban was almost up. But before she could return to competition, she had to undergo three separate drug tests. Antilskaya was on the case.

The first time she turned up at the apartment, Yuliya pressed the record button and didn't waste much time turning the conversation to doping. Too soon. Antilskaya sensed something not right and refused to engage. Yuliya could see her wondering, 'Why is she asking me these questions?' Yuliya blamed herself. Too pushy, too many questions about doping and Melnikov.

With the second test, Yuliya was smarter. She placed her phone on top of the microwave in the kitchen, in plain sight. She again adhered to Vitaly's protocols. Never try to hide the phone; put it where it would normally be. For this test, Antilskaya brought her young son along. Everything was more relaxed. They did the paperwork in the kitchen and Yuliya never mentioned doping. It was Antilskaya who brought up the subject. So amiable was the atmosphere that when Yuliya walked from the kitchen to the bathroom to provide her sample, Antilskaya stayed where she was. All the time, the camera in Yuliya's phone was capturing the doping control officer's utter disregard for the rules.

Vitaly passed the video on to Hajo Seppelt. Antilskaya wasn't important enough to include in the main documentary, but a week or so later German television broadcast a number of shorter pieces, one of which featured her approach to drug testing. Not long after the clip aired, IDTM announced that Ekaterina Antilskaya would no longer be working for the company.

~

They stayed in Seppelt's apartment for a month and a half. Until Seppelt and his mother had had enough of each other and he rang them.

'How are things? Good. Good. Listen, when are you guys moving out?'

'Well, Hajo, I thought that was your part?' Vitaly replied. 'To arrange something for us?'

They didn't want to seem demanding. They had travelled far with Seppelt. He hadn't let them down and had delivered the documentary that would begin a domino effect that would change sport. But a commitment was a commitment. Eventually, a new apartment was found. Bare and unfurnished. Not even a lamp. Not even a bulb. Christoph Kopp was around to help with everything, and life settled down to its new rhythm as WADA, the IAAF and the world of Russian sport engaged in a three-way megaphone battle.

Vitaly's campaign had taken almost seven years to wage. Seven years since he'd joined Rusada, hoping to be an untouchable. The meetings, the calls, so many carefully composed emails and letters, the promises, the offers, Jack Robertson moving like an invisible hand. And all the time holding a family together that included a wife living deep within the system. He knew that the only people who might be grateful for what they had done were the ones who would say nothing. The silent tribe of clean athletes. Anyone not happy or merely pretending to be happy was a stakeholder with territory to protect.

In New York, a lifetime ago, one of Vitaly's college assignments had been to memorise some lines from a movie that he liked. There was only one choice for Vitaly. In a place downtown he'd found a copy of the *Forrest Gump* script. Other students made choices that made them appear more cerebral or that allowed them to comically overact. They never knew when an assignment would turn out to be a casting call for Hollywood. For Vitaly, though, Gump had always resonated. Often, like Gump, he felt like a fool and a stammering outsider. His only armour was telling the truth and being straightforward. Don't try to be smart, he told himself, just be yourself. When you die they don't give out bonus points for how well you kidded people.

Every place Vitaly had been, he had found good people and bad people. The Markowitzes offered kindness that didn't recognise borders. Christoph Kopp did the same. No one place had a monopoly on good or bad. When people asked him if it was worth it, he always said that it was better to have fought well with honour and to have lost than it was to have cheated and won. Why? Well, in the end nobody wins. Would the meek inherit the earth, though? Only if they got it nailed down in writing. Somebody needed to get out there and fight for the clean and meek and their sport. That was his version of running across America.

~

An email came from Yuliya's contact at the Russian police, concerning her employment. There was a difficulty. Could they talk? So early in the New Year Yuliya turned on her mobile for the phone call.

'Where are you? What is happening? We have to fire you.'

She handed the phone over to Vitaly.

'Why are you firing my wife exactly? Because she is trying to fight for the right thing!'

'No, just because she is not competing. If she doesn't compete at the National Indoors in February we will have to fire her.'

'Well, she may be there.'

'Oh. Okay, then.'

Vitaly returned the phone to Yuliya, who promptly switched it off.

The National Indoors came and went. Another email. Another prearranged phone call.

'I'm afraid that the Russian Athletics Federation called us and said that we must fire your wife.'

'So this is how it works,' said Vitaly, 'the Russian Athletics Federation tells the police what to do. That is nice to know!'

Yuliya wrote a letter to the police athletics department, resigning before they could fire her. Vitaly couldn't let the letter go without adding a postscript wondering what the police would say when the inevitable investigation began and it was revealed that police coaches and athletes were involved in drugs, the possession and import of which were criminal offences in Russia.

No reply.

~

After ten months they moved on. It was September 2015. The next chapter needed to begin.

Threats were being made on their lives in Germany. They were constantly aware of the hatred coming at them from the flamethrower of public opinion in Russia. Never far from their thoughts either was the list of dead men and women who had died mysterious, agonising or bizarre deaths after calling out Russia and its sins. That list was bloated by the names of those disappeared, presumed dead.

They were both glad to be moving on.

In Germany there were many times when Yuliya had felt very

scared. She would wake up at night, thinking she had heard movement in the apartment. Somebody had been sent from Russia to kill them. They lived and trained in Marzahn, in what was once the eastern side of Berlin. The area was home to too many Russians. She would hear Russian spoken on German streets. On Fridays she'd notice some of her compatriots making an early start to their weekend drinking. Sometimes as she pushed the pram and carried the groceries, she would hear arguments in Russian from high windows and balconies. They kept themselves to themselves, never once pining for home.

To have some hope for the future, she needed to feel like a real athlete still. To do so, she needed to maintain her file on the online ADAMS system for WADA. It was agreed that access to her ADAMS details, and most especially to her whereabouts, would be accessible only to two people: one from WADA and one from the IAAF. One day Vitaly checked her file. It had been accessed by Rusada, IDTM and Russian Athletics. They knew where she was.

Vitaly found it hard at times like this not to feel some ambivalence towards WADA. The doping police were long on encouragement and short on action. While they were having conferences and dinners, Russia had been hoodwinking them for years. At times they had appeared more interested in Yuliya than in what Yuliya's story could offer them. And now his family's security had been compromised because their system was about as safe as a chicken coop with a flap entrance for foxes. He wrote an emotional letter to WADA and the IAAF, asking if they might publish the addresses and daily movements of Sebastian Coe and WADA president Craig Reedie.

In Marzhan their main security precaution was that the buzzer for their apartment had the common German name Mueller written beside it. *Not really enough, is it*, Yuliya thought. *Russia does doping well, but no better than it does assassination.*

~

These days, Yuliya runs most days in the American sunshine under the blue skies that Vitaly had always yearned for. She has regrets. How could she not, she says at first? But as life moves on, she has a sense that hers was a destiny foretold. It was meant to be. Mistakes and heartaches and troubles.

When most of Russia would have let her swing from a rope, when guilty athletes threatened to sue her until she bled, when Mokhnev claimed she was a traitor who had done this to Russia because he, Mokhnev, would not marry her . . . there was one voice absent from the chorus. Mariya Savinova said nothing. Her silence was dignified. And a mercy. Yuliya hopes often that Mariya will be okay, that the baby she has had will fill her life with the same joy that Robert brought. And that maybe one day she will understand.

Regrets. Like all the time Yuliya lost, being a fool to herself and a liar to Vitaly. If she could erase it all she would. She misses her family but not Kursk. Her family first heard of the entire adventure when news trickled through to Kursk four or five days after Seppelt's film. They had assumed she was in Chelyabinsk with her son and her weird, non-drinking, non-dancing husband. Her son who had been born in Chelyabinsk.

They'd had no goodbyes.

When she has a chance now she talks to them on Skype. For a while she also stayed in contact with Zina, her old friend from Kursk, but Zina never really understood. 'Everybody dopes,' Zina would say, 'so what was the point of doing what you did?'

When Yuliya thinks of doping now, it seems like another life. She recalls the feeling, vaguely, the aggression she felt, the confidence she had that she would be faster. She would be lying if she said that running didn't give her more pleasure when she ran faster. She understands for the first time since she was a kid back in Kursk that she can run without pharma. She still goes out and she does her intervals and she thinks, *Look, girl. Yes, you can run.* She still dreams she will end up running in the Olympics. The happiness is profound and the worry is gone. She knows the pleasure of blue, cloudless skies.

The ripples of Seppelt's documentary and the investigation it caused will be felt in her life for a long, long time to come. For ever, maybe. But she is at peace with it all. The hate that seeps from her homeland doesn't bother her. She was wrong. Then she was right. She was lost. Then she was found.

Often Vitaly has to travel. When he is gone for a day or two and she is alone with Robert, she notes a surprising feeling within her. She misses her husband. *I love him. He loves me. I help him, and he helps me. If he travels without us, I worry about him.*

And she checks the ground between her feet lest she is dreaming.

Epilogue

When Vitaly and Yuliya first considered becoming whistle-blowers they didn't know the meaning of the word. Nor could they imagine the scale of the fallout from their actions. Olympic and World Championship medals would be stripped, world records vacated, bans handed out, reputations lost. The collective memory of events like the 2012 summer Olympics in London and the 2014 Winter Games in Sochi would henceforth be seen through the cloud of Russia's state-organised cheating. Through the Olympics of 2016 in Rio – and even the Tokyo Games, whenever they might happen – the reverberations have become part of the story. Correcting what had gone wrong with Russian sport is a project that will require long and continuous attention.

They lit a fuse, and the explosion that followed would reach backwards and forwards in time. Meanwhile, Vitaly and Yuliya had lives to live and a child to raise.

~

From his first meeting with the Stepanovs, Hajo Seppelt had believed in the story. The more he had got to know them, the surer he had felt. He was in a studio in Cologne when he saw his own completed documentary for the first time. After all his work, Seppelt was downcast: 'I thought it was boring.' He had become the chef who could no longer taste the food he was preparing.

At their offices in Montreal's Stock Exchange Tower, WADA waited to see what Seppelt's film would bring. Though the agency hadn't been able to go after Russia, its investigator Jack Robertson had been matchmaker in the Stepanov–Seppelt production. In a way, the film was also his baby. They had a sense of what was coming; Seppelt had visited Montreal to interview senior WADA figures. President Craig Reedie told staff to wait and see. This might be containable. He knew the sports minister Vitaly Mutko and was hopeful the fallout wouldn't have to be played out in public.

In a sports world battered by wave after wave of scandal, *Top Secret Doping – How Russia Makes Its Winners* was a bona fide tsunami. Seppelt thought he'd known what to expect. 'I was blown away by the reaction. Never in my working life had I been involved in anything that echoed like this.'

Vitaly and Yuliya's evidence was damning. Voice-authentication technology could have been used to verify the secret recordings. Russia never asked for that. Seppelt had tracked down other witnesses. Yevgeniya Pecherina (a former discus thrower serving a ten-year doping ban) alleged that 99 per cent of Russian athletes were doping. The 2010 London Marathon winner Liliya Shobukhova claimed she paid the Russian Athletics Federation €450,000 to cover up a positive test.

Reedie's hope that matters could be resolved over a glass of red never stood much of a chance. On 16 December, thirteen days after the documentary, WADA announced that an independent commission, chaired by Canadian lawyer Dick Pound, had been set up.

Jack Robertson was pleased. For three years, he'd been frustrated by the lack of support from within WADA. Every time he'd asked for additional investigators, he was told there was no money. When extra funding turned up, every department but his got new staff. It wasn't uncommon for Robertson to be first into WADA's offices and last to leave. Long shifts didn't help the throat cancer he has developed. Speaking became difficult but, in an interview with journalist David Epstein, he spelled out his motivations.

'For all of my career I ran informants and whistle-blowers, and every time I had to determine what their motivation was for co-operating. Some for revenge, some for money, some for lighter punishments, some to atone for sins. In my thirty-plus years in investigations, I have never ever met two people that had more pure motives than Yuliya and Vitaly.'

In the days after Seppelt's documentary, Robertson worried that Reedie would try to ride out the storm. After speaking with the agency's director general, David Howman, the chief investigator suggested to people at the United States Anti-Doping Agency that they write to Reedie and press him to launch an investigation. By then the WADA president was already committed to investigating.

Pound's report was delivered in November 2015. It was a blow. Eight months later came the haymaker, a WADA-backed report delivered by another Canadian lawyer, Richard McLaren. Pound's report was damning. McLaren's was coruscating. Everything the Stepanovs alleged turned out to be true.

In Russia the reaction was predictable. The Stepanovs became instant targets. They were denounced and vilified. Vitaly contacted a journalist from *Sovetsky Sport* and offered an interview in the hope of creating a better understanding. That wasn't how it worked out. After publication, a reporter from *Sovetsky Sport* called up Minister Mutko for reaction. The response was perfectly in tune with Russia's attitude – official and unofficial – to Vitaly and Yuliya.

'I know your newspaper for a long time,' Mutko said. 'This is your work. Possibly this is your priority. Why do you treat your home country like dirt?'

In April 2015 Craig Reedie emailed Natalia Zhelanova, the woman appointed by Mutko to take charge of Russia's anti-doping affairs. WADA's president helpfully suggested that what was shown in the documentary was based on practices that pre-dated greater investment in Russian anti-doping. More than that, Reedie asked Zhelanova to pass on his best wishes to her boss.

'On a personal level I value the relationship I have with Minister Mutko and I shall be grateful if you will inform him that there is no intention in WADA to do anything to affect that relationship.'

No such warmth was extended to the Stepanovs.

Former IAAF treasurer and former president of the Russian Athletics Federation, Valentin Balakhnichev, dismissed their evidence as 'anti-Russian propaganda'. Andrei Mitkov, editor of the website allsportinfo.ru, suggested the people supporting the Stepanovs could be connected to the doping mafia whose real intention was to take advantage of the huge Russian doping black market. Yevgeny Trofimov, coach to double Olympic champion pole-vaulter Yelena Isinbayeva, wondered aloud where the media found such naive and unintelligent people as the Stepanovs. Olympic high-jump champion from the 2008 Games in Beijing, Andrey Silnov, went further: 'I can tell them one thing: let them giggle around the corner, enjoy the decision, which they made. I can directly call them traitors who left and gave all kinds of information there. They said all kinds of non-sense. The traitors were always shot first in the war. Therefore, you yourself can draw conclusions.'

After Pound's report, Minister Mutko again turned the flamethrower on the messengers. Yuliya in particular.

'I always try to think well of people but there is a term "stool pigeon" in the anti-doping code.'

～

The Stepanovs understood now what it meant to be whistle-blowers. They knew enough of their country's history to know that being publicly denounced from within the Kremlin was the beginning of a process that stood no chance of ending in reconciliation and a good chance of ending in assassination. In Russia they were branded as traitors. In other places they were considered problematic. They had no plan and nowhere to go. They fell back on each other for strength, focused on Robert and those things that brought serenity.

The line of dominoes they had upset continued to topple. Following the publication of Pound's report, the IAAF banned the Russian Athletics Federation. WADA declared the Russia anti-doping agency non-compliant. No one outside of Russia thought the sanctions harsh. In Moscow, Mr Mutko needed to acknowledge that mistakes had been made.

Grigory Rodchenkov was still head of Moscow's anti-doping laboratory. Mutko told him that heads would have to roll. Where better to start, Mutko felt, than with Rodchenkov's own head? And that of Nikita Kamaev, head of the anti-doping agency. Two heads might be sufficient sacrifice to appease the baying critics.

Rodchenkov was offered a new bureaucratic role. He would rather have walked barefoot to Siberia. He defected to the US and hid in plain sight by telling everything he knew, which was a lot. From his homeland he had taken computer files with details of the bodies and where they were buried. Rodchenkov advised Kamaev to get out of Russia. His friend had a different plan, however. Kamaev knew his time at the agency was up. In early December his exit from Rusada would be confirmed and he would be asked to step down as a member of the medical commission of cycling's governing body, Union Cycliste Internationale (UCI). His career in anti-doping was over.

On 21 November 2015 Kamaev sent an email to the sports department of the *Sunday Times* in London.

'Good evening,' it said. 'Can I ask for Mr Walsh's email for personal conversation?'

Kamaev wrote to me the next day.

> Dear Mr Walsh,
>
> I am writing because you are a reputable person in the field of sports journalism and anti-doping issues.
>
> I want to write a book about the true story of sport pharmacology and doping in Russia since 1987 while being a young scientist working in secret lab in USSR Institute of Sports Medicine. Recent anti-doping controversies prompted me to write the memories associated with both my scientific studies and work in Rusada from 2010.
>
> I have the information and facts that have never been published. I am looking for a co-author to work on a book . . . are you interested?
>
> Best regards,
> Nikita Kamaev
> Executive Director, Russian Anti-doping Agency

On 3 December, I replied.

> Dear Mr Kamaev,
>
> I am interested in helping you to write your book and I might well be able to help find a publisher, certainly in the UK. I would need to be sure that you intend to be 100% honest in the story that you tell and that we would have enough material to produce an engaging, informative and important book. Are you prepared to reveal all that you have learned since 1987? If you do speak English, perhaps we could have a Skype call.
>
> Best regards,
> David Walsh

He soon followed up.

> Dear Mr Walsh,
>
> My personal archive contains actual documents, including confidential sources, regarding the development of performance-enhancing drugs and medicine in sport, correspondence with the anti-doping community, ministry of sports, IOC, NOC, WADA, personally and more.
>
> I apologise for my barbaric poor English, but I'll try my best to be understood.
>
> Skype (kamaev_nikita.) is a good option.
>
> Ready to chat next week.
>
> Very best regards,
>
> Nikita

I worried about how deeply embedded in the system Kamaev had been and about the difficulties posed by his 'barbaric poor English'. We never got round to that Skype call, however. On 14 February 2016, less than three months after writing to the *Sunday Times*, Nikita Kamaev was found dead. It was announced that he'd had a heart attack. He was fifty-two. That morning he'd been cross-country skiing. Reports claimed he experienced chest pain after his exercise and died suddenly.

Eleven days earlier, the man he'd replaced at Rusada, Vyacheslav Sinev had died. Sinev was fifty-seven. He was diabetic. Former Rusada director general Ramil Khabriev told the BBC that Sinev had been waiting for a heart transplant.

Grigory Rodchenkov wrote an opinion piece for the *New York Times* in which he suggested that Nikita Kamaev was assassinated by authorities who'd learned that he was planning to write a book. Rodchenkov also claimed that two days before he himself defected, an insider had warned him that the government was planning his 'suicide'. *Pravda*, no less, quoted Yuri Ganus, the new head of Rusada, as saying the deaths of his predecessors Sinev and Kamaev were suspicious.

'It's clear that two people could not just die like this,' Ganus said. 'I do not have any facts, and as a lawyer I can say that until the opposite is proven I cannot say anything. I understand there was a situation, and the entire anti-doping organisation was disqualified, and in this regard, this [the two deaths] is an extraordinary fact.'

∼

Vitaly, Yuliya and Robert Stepanov had left Germany on 10 September 2015. They landed at Hartsfield–Jackson airport in Atlanta. The dream was a new life in America. The reality would turn out to be two Russian refugees seeking asylum in the US. Kindnesses came to them in small, good ways. Help with finding a place to stay, advice on where to run, coaching, crowdfunding. Soon after the documentary, Travis Tygart, chief executive of the United States Anti-Doping Agency, reached out and offered his backing. Tygart has been steadfast in his support for the couple.

Swiss-born Patrick Magyar got in touch. He'd founded the Diamond League in 2009 and organised the European Championships as well as running his own marketing company. He would become a pillar in their lives. Magyar set up the crowdfunding appeal that allowed the couple to continue their education in the US. $85,765.12 was contributed. Yuliya began English classes, Vitaly signed up for online university courses. He did a bachelor's degree and then a master's in management and leadership.

They've tried to make themselves at home in the US. Speaking to friends and family in Russia reminds them of how their lives have changed. Once Yuliya called her sister Gelia.

As it happened, Gelia was visiting her friend Lena Goncharova. Yuliya and Lena had been best friends growing up. They hadn't spoken for five or six years. Now Lena talked Yuliya through a list of their old classmates. Who was married, who was still single, who had kids, who had got divorced. Lena joked to Yuliya that if she was kicked out of the US, she could come back to Russia and they'd find a factory for her to work in.

'What do our classmates say about me?' Yuliya asked Lena. 'Do they hate me?'

'When you were in the news, everyone talked about it. Now, they're just getting on with their own lives . . . If anything, they are jealous that you have been able to leave Russia and now live in America. It was in the newspapers here that you were invited to the White House?'

'That wasn't a big deal,' Yuliya said, trying to play it down.

On 25 July 2018, Yuliya spoke at a senate hearing in Washington, organised by the Commission on Security and Cooperation in Europe, also known as the Helsinki Commission. Three months earlier Rodchenkov had spoken to the Commission of his experiences inside the Russian doping system.

On 31 October 2018 came the invitation to the White House. With Vitaly, she prepared the words she would say. From a first, tentative date between a doped athlete and an anti-doping tester to jointly writing a speech for a visit to the White House was quite the journey.

'Hello, I am Yuliya Stepanova,' she began. 'Thank you for inviting me to be here. I would like to begin by apologising about my doping past. Unfortunately, I cannot change my past. As an athlete, I was a part of the Russian doping system, I cheated, and now I am talking about it. For the past six years, as a whistle-blower, I am trying to show that I changed and now help make sports clean.'

She recalled the milestones of her athletics career: first competition, aged seventeen; first doping (testosterone), aged twenty; through courses of anabolic steroids and erythropoietin. She told her audience that erythropoietic treatments meant iron supplementation and that now her iron levels are twenty times higher than they should be, an anomaly she can control these days through intense exercising.

At the end of her short talk, Yuliya concluded, 'I am glad to be here, and it feels that standing up for the right reasons is more rewarding than winning medals. Thank you.' She recalls the standing ovation with some wonder. 'I just felt so uncomfortable. Why are you clapping?'

Since moving to the US, she has discovered things about herself. She has been surprised. Before the 2016 Rio Games, there was an online campaign calling for the IOC to invite her to compete as one of the 'neutral' athletes. The petition attracted 274,215 signatures. Vitaly and Patrick Magyar encouraged her. She felt differently. There was a nagging foot injury, and deep down she just wasn't that bothered.

'One day I was thinking about why some people can be Olympic champions and some cannot be. My opinion is that some want it more than others.'

She still runs. 'For my health; it's for my body and for my mind. If I do a good run, I feel very good afterwards.' The focus of the professional athlete is gone, though. She can scarcely imagine it. 'I don't want to live for just sport and achieving results. I've let that go.'

One day at a fitness centre Yuliya met Amanda, another runner who was also nursing a minor injury. They got talking. Amanda invited Yuliya to a Bible-study group that her friend Mark organised. At the first meeting, Mark introduced Yuliya to the group. He asked if she missed Russia and were there times when she longed to be back home?

'Before, that is when I was in Russia, I never felt at home. It was like my soul was somewhere else. Vitaly and I lived in different places and always I thought this is not the place I'd like to spend the rest of my life. In America I feel like I am at home.'

The girl who once sat in a room in Kursk captivated by Cathy Freeman at the Sydney Olympics has changed.

～

On 1 January 2009, Vitaly signed up on the website RunningAHEAD, which allowed him to log his daily runs. Posting his numbers encouraged him to keep running, if only to enjoy the satisfaction of another entry. His aim was to run every day of his life.

'Mama always said stupid is as stupid does,' is one of his favourite *Forrest Gump* lines. Not because he thinks the hero of the movie is unintelligent but rather because the fixation on running seemed stupid to Vitaly. Forrest Gump ran for three years, two months, fourteen days and sixteen hours. What kind of simpleton would keep running that long? Vitaly's statistics on RunningAHEAD speak of the same madness. His longest unbroken sequence was 412 days, during which he covered 6,629.9 kilometres, or a daily average of 16.1 kilometres for one year, one month and seventeen days. In the eleven years and three months since he began recording his runs, he has covered 46,517 kilometres at an average pace of 4:54 per kilometre. To put this another way, if he had decided to run around the circumference of the Earth, he would now be on his second lap.

There is another *Forrest Gump* quote he thinks about: 'I don't know if we each have a destiny, or if we're all just floatin' around, accidental-like on a breeze, but I, I think maybe it's both.' Vitaly wonders if it was his destiny to end up at Rusada or whether it was all just the weirdest accident.

He sees himself as the simpleton who thought he could save something precious, just like the Dutch boy who put his finger in the dyke and saved his country. Vitaly resists any notion of being a saviour but, noting that Russia is now banned from international competition, he senses that things have changed and will continue to do so.

~

America has brought new lives and better memories. None better than a weekend spent in the antebellum glory of Savannah, Georgia. Sharon Kelley, a friend they made at an anti-doping conference, invited them to Tampa, Florida, to speak at another conference. As their friendship grew, Kelley asked them to Savannah for her birthday party and covered the cost of their trip. They relaxed by the hotel swimming pool with Robert, they went to watch dolphins, they caught shrimp. On the boat Robert got to see the shrimp close up.

Kelley also arranged a bus tour of the city. Yuliya was keen. Robert would have fun, wouldn't he? Vitaly was doubtful. In the sweltering heat and soupy humidity, a city tour? This was 14 August 2018. He resisted but it was futile. He had lost bigger battles to Yuliya in the past and now he surrendered gracefully.

Arriving at the Old Town Trolley Tour pick-up point, they just missed an outgoing tour. Even waiting twenty minutes in the shade, they overheated. Vitaly's silence told Yuliya he might not forgive her for this. When another trolley came, the seats were fake leather and painfully hot. Yuliya and Robert didn't complain. They hopped off at the Pirate's House, a landmark attraction in Savannah, and Yuliya thought it the coolest place she'd ever seen. They ate there and picked up another trolley to complete the tour.

By the time they got to Chippewa Square, Vitaly was barely listening to the tour guide any more. In the background to his thoughts and sweat, a voice mentioned that the square was a favourite location for Hollywood film-makers.

'And this is where Forrest Gump sat and told his story to anyone who would listen while waiting for a bus.'

Vitaly was alive again. He gazed down at a scene that was as familiar to him as any place he had grown up in. How many times had he watched those opening moments, that feather floating through the credits towards this actual spot to be plucked from the ground by a man in a pale suit and old runners who would place it carefully in his battered briefcase? The original bench, a movie prop, now rested in the Savannah History Museum, but just to be on this square, breathing the same thick air and seeing the same elegant sights, felt to Vitaly like a fulfilment.

He glanced at Yuliya. She was smiling.

Not every day has been that perfect. Vitaly and Yuliya struggle on. They try not to stress about what the US is going to do with them. For now, their fate still rests in the hands of others.

I asked Vitaly once why it all meant so much, this crusade, this passion, this tilting at windmills.

'It's obvious,' he said. 'In the end we all die and nobody wins. Why not try to leave a good mark?'

Vitaly and Yuliya continue to run every day. Robert is six now and fluent in English and Russian. His parents have so many stories to tell him when the time comes. As of now, many of those stories still remain unfinished.

Appendix 1

11 October 2010
Email from Vitaly Stepanov to Stuart Kemp of WADA

Dear Stuart, how are you?

I'm sorry I didn't write to you earlier. I guess there was a lot going on and I didn't really understand where everything is going. Well, I still don't understand a lot of things. But I did decide that I will stay on your (WADA code) side and let you know what I know and hopefully it will help you with your decisions. I'm not gonna hide any names or any information from you, even though I do realise that my opinion might be a lot different from other opinions that you are getting from Russia.

The only solution I see at this point is to have WADA independent observers (people you can really trust) to stay in Russia at all the time and check how everything is being done.

Or you have to find people in Russia that you can trust and somehow help them to be in charge of the lab and the nado [National Anti-Doping Organisation].

I have three different stories for you that are all related

to the anti-doping field: my story, Rusada's story and my wife's story.

I'll begin with the toughest one.

My wife, RUSANOVA Yuliya, is not in the IAAF registered testing pool. There is no such thing as the national registered testing pool as of now. So, just like most of the other Russian athletes, she is being tested only after big national competitions or while she is on the training camp with the Russian national team.

Just like any other athlete, she has a dream of competing at the Olympics and, just like any other female professional athlete competing at track events in Russia, she realises that the only way to get to the Olympics is by doping.

If you put it in times – without doping she runs 2:05; with doping she runs 1:59. To qualify for the Olympics you would probably have to run in about 1:57 twice in two days. I'm not trying to make excuses for the way she thinks and she does, but I do hope that I won't be the one who breaks her dreams.

Let me tell you how her summer season went and how she achieved those results.

Her coach buys doping from a person who knows Grigory Rodchenkov very well. So some of the money that is being paid for doping goes to Grigory.

All the coaches plan the preparation of athletes for the events by using information that is being provided by Grigory. The information includes the doses that can be used and how long it takes to clean up (so it doesn't show in urine samples). Most of the coaches don't tell athletes what they are giving to them. There is also another way that Grigory makes money. Some coaches (not all) that know him personally can call him directly right after the sample was taken and tell him the dirty sample code number, and for $300 he would make sure that positive sample wouldn't come out. If the sample was analysed but the official results were not sent out yet he can still hide the sample, only the price for this is $1,000.

My wife didn't do as well as she was hoping during the winter season. So her coach had to make some changes during the preparation for the summer season. A few months before the main competition, the course of steroids is being done, after that EPO, testosterone, and human growth hormone. Grigory tells the coaches that the last dose of EPO must be eight to ten days before the start. I don't understand most of the medical terminologies but I believe that there are two types of EPO that Russian athletes use:

Epocrinum (Epoetin alfa), which is possible to buy in Russian pharmacies, and another type of EPO. The other type seems to have bigger effects. Supposedly it is some kind of Japanese EPO that was somehow modified by the lab in Moscow region (I don't know where it is exactly located) and the ampoule with this kind of EPO just says 'water II'. I was even told that supposedly European labs can't detect such EPO. I just want to mention once again that I don't know if the information I'm giving to you is 100 per cent correct but it does make sense at least to me.

My wife had to use the 'water II' type EPO for the first time this year as the course of Epocrinum wasn't getting her haemoglobin higher. Supposedly the Epocrinum she used went bad and she had to use something stronger to try to still have a good time at the competitions. After a few doses of 'water II' her haemoglobin jumped from

140 to 187. I hope you do realise that it's not easy for me to provide this information to you. During the past six months or so I keep wondering how I could get myself in such situation. And well, I guess everything happens for a reason and if you want to battle something you have to at least know what you are battling.

So at the end of May there were qualifying competitions in Sochi for European Team Championships. Unexpectedly my wife won the 800 metres and her sample was clean. But she didn't go to the Team Championships because the coach from Moscow (Styrkina) told the national team coach that they have to take her athlete (Svetlana Klyuka) if they don't want any problems. Styrkina is one of the coaches that works directly with Grigory. So my wife didn't compete at the European Team Championships, but she was noticed. Then her coach had a few talks with the coach (Melnikov) from the national team. I guess those talks didn't go well at some point. My guess is that Mr Melnikov didn't like that my wife's coach (Mr Mohnev [sic]) doesn't tell Mr Melnikov how my wife was being prepared. So in July there was Russian Athletics Championships (qualifiers for European Championships in Barcelona). My wife finished third in 800 and fifth in 1500 metres. She was satisfied with those results even though she didn't qualify for the European Championships. Right after the Championships in Barcelona one of the coaches (while being drunk) called Mr Mohnev and told him that supposedly my wife's sample was positive (EPO and steroids). I don't know if the sample was positive or not but Mr Mohnev paid to the person from whom he buys doping $1,000. The next morning Grigory

Rodchenkov called Mr Mohnev and explained that this kind of EPO can be only detected by the Moscow lab and can't be detected by other labs, but the last dose should have been ten days before the test. Previously Mr Mohnev said that the last dose was eight days before the test. And since Mr Mohnev didn't call Grigory before the sample was analysed, he had to pay $1,000 (not $300). This whole story somewhat doesn't make sense but that is how it happened and it shows that the whole system is very corrupt. I tried to make this story short but of course in person I could tell you the more detailed version. During this whole situation I stayed away from it and just looked from the side how everything turns out. Mr Mohnev and Mr Melnikov will meet in a week or so to try to have a good conversation about my wife's future. Mr Melnikov is the one who is responsible for making sure that all middle- and long-distance runners are clean while being tested. He is the one who helps Mr Chegin's walkers as well.

So, this is my wife's story. She is very talented and self-motivated and I do believe that she could achieve a lot by competing clean if the competition was clean as well.

Rusada story
I'll just make some points (all of the points that are below in the previous letters are true as well):

1. the testing – it's only getting worse – most of the testing is being done with advance notice.

– the directors don't really care about who is being tested and we have young girls responsible for planning and the only thing they care about is to get enough samples by the end of the month.

— a lot of times our DCOs come to do testing and take sample from any athletes they can find at the training camp. This is true for blood passport as well.

2. Igor Zagorskiy is flying to Canada this week but it seems that he said something wrong somewhere as the people from the ministry don't like him a lot and believe that he is giving some kind of secret information to WADA. Mr Virupaev thinks that Igor had to provide some kind of secret information in order to become a member of WADA education committee.

3. Also Mr Virupaev mentioned that he is being annoyed by constant substitution (tampering) of samples by ARAF. I don't know exactly what he meant but that's what he told me.

4. I still do DCO training but for the last three new DCOs our training was being done in five hours. This is how much our directors give me to do the training. Even though I believe to all IFs and to WADA we tell that the urine sample collection training is being done in three days.

5. In June I was told to make Rusada DCO manual. But the whole point of it was to try to make sure that I won't be able to do it the right way (as there was no right way), so they can fire me. At the end of their try there was a ten-page DCO manual (instead of original eighty as it was in WADA manual) signed by Vyacheslav Sinev and for the past three months this document is not being used at all. None of our old DCOs had a recertification in 2010.

6. You know, at some point all you can do at work is laugh. While Mr Fahey was in Russia, Mr Sinev presented to him the Russian version of 'Always Picked Last'. I still write emails to Jennifer to get the official permission to print this book. But we were told to print it and publish it in July as we had to show something new for the forum.

7. Today people at work were saying that Igor Zagorskiy and Natalya Govorkova (financial director) are going to leave Rusada in November. As they are the ones that are mostly disliked by the ministry. Of course this information is not official.

8. Nobody is doing anything about ISO. In general, the ministry doesn't like that Rusada is working closely with Antidoping Norway as Russia shouldn't be providing any information of how we do things in Russia. The ministry, not WADA, should decide who should be punished for doping and who should be able to use doping to get the medals.

9. It seems that all four of our directors are on their own. They almost don't talk to each other and it looks that each one separately is just trying to stay for as long as possible at Rusada. Mr Khabriev doesn't come to Rusada often (two to three times per week for a few hours).

My story
Our directors keep trying to get rid of me, but not doing it as hard as in the beginning of the summer. I mostly do education seminars for different federations. Any travels abroad are prohibited for me and the

directors keep showing me any way possible that I'm useless. I keep running and I will probably do another Boston marathon in 2011. In November for my vacation I'm going to a training camp to Kislovodsk to run with my wife. If it weren't for you I would have left Rusada already, but for some reason I believe that WADA is made for the right cause and I really do hope I can battle doping and be on your side. Although I do realise that the faster my wife gets, the harder for you it would be to communicate to me. I do hope there are non-prohibited ways to get her as fast as she is now or may be even faster. So, if there was a way to move to a different country and see how things are being done there, I would try to get her to move. But as of now it seems like an impossible dream.

Sorry that the letter is so long.

And I hope you get some helpful information from it. I trust you, so I don't mind if you show this letter to other WADA people.

You can be sure that from my side there won't be any double games and you can contact me any time just in case you need any kind of information.

I hope all is well in your family and WADA.

Please, let me know that you received this letter.

Best regards,

Vitaly

Draft emails from Vitaly Stepanov to Stuart Kemp

Below are the letters that I wrote to you earlier but never finished it and sent it to you. I just thought that you might get something from it as well.

Letter 1

I guess I really would like to chat personally, but as it is not possible at this moment I'll try to put some of my thoughts on the paper.

1. People from the ministry (I had three long unofficial talks with Konstantin Virupaev, and I believe he was telling me the points that are coming directly from Mr Mutko) and Rusada feel that some information might be leaking to WADA and IFs. As this being said we should be very, very careful. I'm guessing they are somewhat suspicious of me, but they do not have any kind of proof. A few days ago I got an open envelope that was sent from you in March to our old address and I only got it a few days ago and it was open. Please, say thank you to Stacy for sending it. I really appreciate it. I guess it helped me somewhat on one hand, as our directors probably got the idea that maybe they shouldn't try to get rid of me, but on the other hand it got them thinking that I might be connected to you in some way. I'm getting the feeling that they are even checking documents on my desk and work computer while I'm not in the office. But again, they couldn't find anything there as I keep everything at home and send messages to you from different computers away from home.

2. Last week I went to the ministry and had a two-hour talk with Mr Virupaev. He told me a lot of things straightforward. I guess I really would like to have a bigger picture on how things are being done around the world, as I feel I'm getting deeper and deeper on the situation in our country. As you probably already

noticed, I really don't like to play double games but if it's for a good cause I will do that. But again I wish we could chat and I could try to get a better feeling on what your goals really are with our country and countries like ours. But the main points that I got from the ministry are the following:

1. WADA is not really battling doping, it's all politics.
2. All countries and especially Europe are afraid of Russia and try to not let us win any medals anyway possible.
3. Russia will always work by double standards as prohibited list is mostly politics and there is no really bad health consequences for athletes, so our main goal is to make sure that the athletes are clean while competing abroad and to make sure that there are no spies within our field, so Russia can show that Russia is improving and we are really fighting doping.
4. The ministry would only let DCOs take samples to European labs if there would be a possibility for us to test any foreign athletes anytime around the world and analyse it in our lab (Russian). He called it 'cross testing'. Our ministry feels that the rest of the countries work by double standards and this is the way we will always work as this is the only way to win gold medals. I really hope that this is not true, because then . . . well, then I'm guessing I'm just a naive person who believes in fair sport. I do understand that sometimes you have to make compromises, but I really hope WADA's goal is what the code says.

I will write more later. I'm getting more and more information every day and I understand that our country doesn't want people like me to have the knowledge that I'm getting.

Letter 2

Hi Stuart. I never sent you the letter that I meant to send to you earlier. I just had to try to figure out what it is that I am doing, because ... oh well, because of my wife I'm part of the system that is not in line with the WADA code. On one hand I really would love to keep fighting for the fair sport but on the other I'm 100 per cent sure that sport in Russia is not fair and by competing fairly my wife would never get a chance to achieve her dreams. I'm guessing the solution would be to move to a different country that uses non-prohibited novice methods for preparing athletes and see where it could get her ...

Appendix 2

12 January 2011
Email from Vitaly Stepanov to Stuart Kemp of WADA

Hello. I thought that some of the information below might be useful for you or your colleagues. I hope all is well.

In November I spent the whole month with my wife at the training camp in Kislovodsk (about 1,000 metres above sea level). I didn't make it clear the last time, but my wife and her coach (Mr Mokhnev) are from Kursk region, not Moscow or Moscow region. So like I wrote in the previous letter, Mokhnev and Melnikov (the person responsible for doping preparation of athletes at ARAF) were supposed to chat about my wife's future. It turned out the ARAF had been following her progress the past few years and they were just waiting for her coach to start co-operating with them. So, for the 2011 winter season she is one of the three to five runners that are on national team roster for 800 metres and are being prepared directly for European Championships in Europe in early March. Which means that the doping preparation for the chosen ones is moved for two weeks towards the European Championships. Now my wife's coach is buying doping from Mr Portugalov who is connected with Mr Melnikov and Grigory Rodchenkov. Of course it is more expensive to buy steroids, EPO, HGH and testosterone from Mr Portugalov but you get the following advantages:

• You can compete dirty at any events in Russia, including any national championships (in previous years my wife had to be clean during national championships).

• You are never tested by Rusada when you are dirty. (In November, while I was with my wife at the training camp, there was an announcement from the manager (coach Pudov) of that particular national team camp that Rusada is coming in seven days (actually our DCOs came even later, in nine days) and that there are two lists: athletes that will be tested (that are clean) and athletes that will not be tested (that are not clean). Since we don't have a NRTP [National Registered Testing Pool] there is no missed tests or any kind of other penalties for athletes that are not being tested at the camp.

• ARAF helps you when international DCOs come to test. They hide you if you are dirty and they make sure that you are where you supposed to be when you are clean so you are tested. There are different ways that this can be done but of course it all depends on the lab where the sample is going. Mr Portugalov works in the same building with Mr Rodchenkov.

• Your blood and urine samples are being analysed every two to three weeks and the actual doping preparation is being based on those results . . .

    . . . I don't know how my wife will do this season

but it seems that she should do even better than the last year because she is being helped with doping by ARAF. With this being said, I believe that something similar is being done in many Russian sports and also Ukrainian and Belarussian sports. This I'm assuming from my own experience and the talk of athletes at the camp.

The situation at Rusada

In general, it is only getting worse. Our new executive director, Mr Khabriev, doesn't show up at Rusada often and the things are being done the old way. It seems that Derevoedov and Zagorskiy said that Rusada staff doesn't do much and the person to blame for that is Sinev. So I'm guessing this way the two of them are trying to stay at Rusada and continue doing things their way. So, a few days before New Year everyone in Rusada received official notification that Rusada will have a different structure and none of us will have job positions as of 1 March 2011. Some of us might be offered new job positions but we have to be qualified for those positions. The new structure with the requirements for different positions was even placed on our website, but all requirements are very high which means that most of us don't qualify for the positions that we are at right now. I don't really know why this being done but I guess the logical thing is that Mr Khabriev wants to bring his own team and get rid of most of us. Of course I would have done the same thing if I were the new director, but I'm not. I'm not even qualified for the education manager position :-) sometimes things definitely look so unfair by my standards but again nobody said that life is fair. ;-) I'm not crying here and I'm not giving up but it definitely seems that there are not many Russians that believe in the Code as much as I do. But I do hope that you and your colleagues at WADA keep pushing hard and don't give up. Hmm . . . Below are some other points that I put down in the past few months.

• How Russia planned the amount of urine tests for 2011: the ministry sent out official letters to sports federations requesting the amount of samples that each federation would like to have. Then I guess all those numbers are added and this is how the ministry comes up with the number of tests.

• Concerning the blood testing: the new person at Rusada, Nikita Kamaev (he is in the position of financial director right now, as this was the only position open at Rusada in the beginning of December, but the talk in the office is that he has a medical degree and will be involved with athlete passports somehow. He was brought by Ramil Khabriev) told the education department that the Russian lab didn't get the blood accreditation. None of the other people (Zagorskiy, Sinev or Derevoedov) told us anything about that. Supposedly there was a big scandal in the ministry but nothing came out to the media.

• We are now translating the VANOC [Vancouver Organizing Committee] DCO, BCO, chaperone training manuals for Sochi 2014. Zagorskiy tried to get officially these materials from VANOC and the approval for translation but as far as I know he didn't get the approval but told us to do the translation anyways and use it for our purposes.

• Mr Lebedev from Sochi OC doesn't know much about

anti-doping as he visits our seminars to get the basic knowledge.

• Mr Samsonov, the person who was in charge of results management at Rusada in 09 and had the notebook with the sample numbers, died in jail of heart attack in October.

• We have two persons at Rusada that call to federations and ask when they would like Rusada to test their athletes. So we can get the necessary amount of samples in time ;-) sorry for smiling so much. I just don't know what else I can do about that at this point.

• Govorkova, financial director at Rusada, and Zinovieva, chief accountant of Rusada from November. As of now we still don't have a chief accountant.

• Mr Nagornih (the main person for anti-doping at the ministry) used to work at the Sports Ministry of Moscow and he administered (made sure that the lab gets financing) the Moscow lab (not the accredited one). And from the talk of different people the main purpose of that lab was money laundering. Natalia Zhelanova, the one on WADA finance and administration committee, is a daughter of a good friend of Mr Nagornih.

• I did doping controls with a Norwegian DCO in December. I was surprised that Zagorskiy actually asked me to do that (maybe they already decided that I'm only at Rusada until March or maybe they are not being as hard on me because they have bigger problems to deal with). Anyways, there was miscommunication between

Sinev and Mr Melnikov (from ARAF). Sinev didn't tell Melnikov the list of the athletes we would like to test before we came to do the testing on the first day, but still you could clearly tell who was hidden when we went to do the testing on the second day.

I understand that I'm writing a lot of names and it could be confusing but I'm always willing to tell and explain in more details to you any necessary information.

... At the end of December one of my colleagues went with Mr Khabriev to a meeting at the Ministry of Sports where Mr Mutko gave the speech about the outcome of 2010. And there were two things that my colleague noticed that were interesting:

a. One of the speeches was made by the executive director of Russian Medical–biological agency, Mr Uyba, and after the speech Mr Khabriev asked him why the doctors of athletes do not apply for TUEs [Therapeutic Use Exemptions] as much as it is necessary. Mr Uyba answered that they gave out about 300 TUEs this year. So either Mr Uyba had no idea what he was answering or they did give out 300 TUEs. :-). The actual number that Rusada dealt with in 2010 is about thirty.

b. After the official part of the speech of Mutko was done and the media left the room, one of the persons asked Mr Mutko: 'Why don't Russia get rid of doctors that are using doping for preparation as most of them are known?' Mutko answered: 'We got rid of some of them in biathlon and now we don't have any medals this season.'

• It seems that our DCO that went with urine samples to Lausanne this morning had no problems at all at the airport. But of course it was our DCO. As far as I understand, any foreign DCO would still have to notify Rusada about doing doping controls as some of the papers that must be shown at the airport must be stamped by Rusada.

• There are other small things that I could mention if we were chatting but I guess I would just mention one more thing. I'm not making any kind of excuses but sometimes I talk with my wife and I tell her that her health is more important for me than anything else but the fair questions that she asks me: Do you want me to quit running? Do you want me to give up on my dreams?

I can't make her quit and I hope you understand that this doping system was here for the past forty years or so and it might take a lot of time for people to change their mindset and start trying to do things the honest and fair way.

Have a great day.

PS. Just in case, I will be in Boston from April 15th until the 19th.

PPS. It would be good to get some answer from you.

Appendix 3

24 February 2011
Email from Vitaly Stepanov to Stuart Kemp of WADA

Hello, how are you? I hope all is well.

I just decided to send a short update to you. Probably in a while I will write a longer message to you with my thoughts if you would need such message.

As of 1 March I won't work at Rusada any longer. Today I got official notification that there are no job openings for me and I will be fired. I guess I knew that it will happen. I just didn't have the official paper until today.

The structure of Rusada as it seems to me as of now:

Mr Khabriev – executive director – he doesn't show up at Rusada often and he doesn't try to get the full understanding.

Mr Kamaev – the person that Mr Khabriev brought to be in charge of Rusada. He is a good friend of Grigory Rodchenkov as he used to work in the same building with Mr Rodchenkov. He doesn't understand a lot of things yet, even though he tries, so he has to listen to Mr Derevoedov and Mr Zagorskiy and makes decisions based on their opinions.

Zagorskiy and Derevoedov will be under Mr Kamaev

but basically stay in charge of everything that goes on at Rusada.

Mr Sinev I believe received the same notification as I did today. About six other people received such notification today as well.

All of the people that are staying at Rusada were brought by Derevoedov and Zagorskiy.

So it seems that at this point there won't be anyone at Rusada that won't follow them and try to do what the code says. I guess I'm disappointed but again I tried to do my job as good as possible it just was not good enough for Rusada.

My wife is winning everything so far this season and I have a feeling that she will do just as well at the European Championships in Paris in eight days. The only thing she was missing the previous seasons is being a part of ARAF preparation system. I don't think Derevoedov or Zagorskiy realise that I'm communicating to you in any way and they probably think that I won't start talking to you after being fired because of the successes of my wife.

I really would love to keep working in anti-doping field but I guess the only way it can happen is with your support. I'm not asking for your help. I just hope you do realise that I tried my best and I will continue doing so if I somehow get in a position where I can try to change things. And I hope you realise that my wife is willing to compete clean if others were competing clean in Russia. She trusts me and I trust your judgement.

Please send a short reply to me that you received this message.

Have a great day.

Appendix 4

28 February 2011
Email from Vitaly Stepanov to Stuart Kemp of WADA

Hi ... this is the last news ...

In addition to the information I gave you a few days ago. The total number of people that left RUSADA is 18. 9 people, including me, Mr. Sinev, and his son, were not offered any new positions. Mr. Sinev received a special money bonus for staying quiet. 9 other people decided to leave RUSADA as they did not like the new positions that they were offered. One of them is Pavel Khorkin, the person responsible for TUEs at RUSADA. 3 of the people are DCOs.

Below is unofficial information, so I really don't know how true it is:

1. Supposedly one of the employees at Rusada heard private conversation between Mr. Habriev and Mr. Kamaev where they were discussing the next steps of restructure of RUSADA: a. in a few months to get rid of Mr. Zagorskiy and Mr. Derevoedov; b. in 4–5 months get rid of the rest RUSADA employees that were not fired at the end of February, and get the whole new staffing.

This does not seem like something that is possible but well, the way RUSADA does things are very illogical sometimes.

2. Supposedly on Feb 24th the people from federal drug control service of the Russian federation caught Grigory Rodchenkov's wife while she was selling steroids. When Mr. Rodchenkov found out this he got some heart problem and was hospitalized. His secretary told that he is ok but on Feb 25th he did not show up at Russian Football Union conference where he was supposed to be one on the speakers. 2 persons from federal drug control service of the Russian federation called to Rusada common phone number on Friday evening requesting Mr.Sinev's mobile number. They said that our (RUSADA) Lab has a big problem and they have to speak to executive director of RUSADA. So, those people that called didn't even know that the lab and Rusada are not the same organization and that Mr. Sinev is not in charge of Rusada. I know that this sounds crazy but this is what the talk is at Rusada and ARAF. There is nothing about it in the media. May be you have a bigger and better picture as this happened the same day as David Howman's statement was placed on your website.

Anyways as always please send a short reply to me and let me know if you want me to keep you updated on this crazy second point.

Appendix 5

4 April 2011
Email from Stuart Kemp of WADA to Vitaly Stepanov

Hello,

We received an interesting email today, that I've pasted below. Do you know anything about this?

Grigoriy Rodchencov, head of Russian antidoping laboratory, under criminal procedure. 11/03/2011 special agent of Russian anti-narcotic inspection (Ministry of internal affair subsidary) taken for criminal court liability mr Rodchencov and [his] sister, Marina. Subject – illegal steroid storage, commercial distribution, is absolutely evident (artical 234 of Russian Criminal law) After preliminary investigation. Mr Rodchencov make a suisade attempt. Now he is in special clinic. Investigation must be continue after his curation. Russian sport officals truy to 'frooze' this story. If you want chek it – do not hesitate to contact me.

Thanks

Appendix 6

17 June 2012
From Vitaly Stepanov to Stuart Kemp of WADA

Hello

Hi, sorry it took a while for me to answer. I didn't have much internet access lately. Unfortunately, I do not have much to write.

My wife had a very good training camp in March in Portugal but I guess pushed a little too much and didn't start taking days off until early May. So, in early April my wife was injured, all April she ran on painkillers hoping that the leg pain would go away but it didn't happen. So, sadly my wife will not be competing this summer season at all and we will just try to make sure that her leg fully recovers for next seasons.

So, as of now we are not doing any kind of pharma preparation and are not running in June at all.

As for the things that might be interesting to you.

As I wrote to you earlier, Mr Melnikov informed my wife's coach about her may testing almost 45 days in advance. I don't know if I had to do anything with the following but in early may Mr Melnikov called to my wife's coach and said that WADA in addition to blood passport will take urine for EPO. So, it meant that my wife couldn't be tested until she was fully clean. And that date was somewhere between 21 May and 25th. Somewhere close to 20 May Mr Melnikov checked once again with my wife's coach when she can be tested (I could be a day off with the info I'm providing to you right now as I don't have my wife's doping control form with me right now). So it was decided that my wife will be tested in Kursk (about 350 miles away from Moscow) on 24 May.

Appendix 7

25 November 2012
Email from Vitaly Stepanov to Stuart Kemp of WADA

Hello, again. I hope everything is well.

I know that we can see my wife's blood passport results in ADAMS. What I was asking, is there a way to get an advice from an expert? I know that IAAF decides if an athlete should be sanctioned or not. I guess I would like to know, if WADA took a close look at her blood passport, would she be sanctioned as of now or would she be in some kind of 'questionable' list?

My wife didn't talk to Mr Melnikov yet, but her new coach after getting drunk told her that my wife basically has two options right now: she can be officially sanctioned or 'unofficially'.

'Unofficially' supposedly means that she cannot compete for two years, but can keep training and she will not be on official IAAF sanctioned list.

There are some Russian runners that are 'unofficially' sanctioned right now. One of them is Anna Alminova, she also trains in Mr Kazarin's group.

I don't know how IAAF and ARAF work on these issues but I guess if IAAF sanctions all ninety-five Russian athletes it will be a little too much. And I guess somebody decides in ARAF or IAAF the number of athletes that should be officially and 'unofficially' sanctioned.

It really seems that people at ARAF and probably Rusada too did not understand the blood passport results at all (for all athletes). If I understand correctly they still don't understand where this situation is going and they are just hoping that it is not as bad as it looks for them.

Supposedly, Mr Portugalov doesn't want to prepare any athletes any longer. He told Mr Kazarin, that it's getting too dangerous and he is getting too old to keep doing it. And he really doesn't care how much more money he can make, because he already has enough.

I guess I will write more in a few weeks after I see where my wife's situation is going.

Thank you for sending my application letter to your colleagues. I actually wanted to write to Rune, Stacy and Olivier a small note sometime later this week to say that I mentioned their names in my application. Could you please give me their correct email addresses? The official application deadline is 2 December.

Do you know why there is a job opening in education department? Did somebody leave WADA? I thought that it might be a good idea to write to Rob as well, but I don't want to be too 'pushy' (as I tend to be this way when I really want something).

Anyways, thank you for taking your time reading this and as always please reply something.

Have a great day.

Notes

Chapter 2

1   In July 2008 Lysenko was found to have tested positive for a hormone blocker. She received a two-year ban, and a world record she had set in 2007 was erased from the records. In February 2019 she received an eight-year ban from sport for doping. The ban was backdated to July 2016, when it emerged on retesting that she had submitted a positive test at the London Olympics in 2012, where she had won the gold medal. She was retrospectively disqualified and stripped of her medal, which she refused to return. She married her coach, Nikolai Beloborodov.

2   In May 2007 Yekaterina Khoroshikh tested positive for methylandrostenediol and was subsequently handed a two-year ban from sport.

3   This record was beaten a year later by Gulfiya Khanafeyeva. Having served a three-month doping ban, it was announced in July 2008 that Khanafeyeva was among seven Russian Olympians who had tested positive. In October 2008 she received a two-year ban for manipulating drug samples. In 2017 she was disqualified from the 2012 Olympics and had her results annulled after retesting yielded a positive. She received an eight-year ban in February 2019.

4   Vitaly had come to Moscow to study sports management. He had promised his parents that – whatever else he did – he would not quit the course. He was done with quitting. In college one of his lecturers had been the noted sports psychologist Rudolf Zagainov. The story went that in the 2002 Winter Olympics at Salt Lake City, Zagainov's cold stare had intimidated the figure skater Evgeni Plushenko so badly that the world champion had just lost his nerve and let Zagainov's man Alexei Yagudin take the gold medal. Vitaly liked the old guy, though. He had worked with thirty-eight world champions. His clients included nineteen Olympic champions. His lectures were always interesting. Vitaly sent Zagainov the occasional note saying as much and offering to work for him if a vacancy arose. Nothing came of it and time passed. Then in the summer of 2007 Zagainov became famous again, when his professional and personal relationship with the European champion track cyclist Yulia Aroustamova came to a sad end. The

354

young woman hanged herself in the flat they had shared together. Yulia was twenty-four. Zagainov was sixty-seven.

Around the same time, another long-running show reached a finale. In July the great hero of Russian biathlon, Alexander Tikhonov, who had retired with eleven world-championship gold medals and four Olympic golds, was found guilty of conspiracy to murder Aman Tuleyev, the governor of the Kemerovo Oblast. Tikhonov was sentenced to three years' imprisonment. That was the bad news. The good news followed immediately: as a national hero, Tikhonov was granted an amnesty and was free to go to lunch. The hero's close friend, Leonid Tyagachev, president of the Russian Olympic Committee, commended the decision of the Novosibirsk Court as soon as the amnesty was confirmed. 'The person who has devoted all his life to Russia can't be guilty in anything,' Tyagachev said, surprising even those citizens with just a passing interest in jurisprudence. Tyagachev said he looked forward to working with Tikhonov in advance of the Sochi Games.

Chapter 7

1   A most notorious case of *dedovshchina* happened near Vitaly's home of Chelyabinsk at the Tank Academy in 2006. Andrei Sychev from Yekaterinburg was just eighteen and hauntingly eager to do his service as his father and grandfather before him had done. Poor Andrei trusted the army. Two days into his draft time in the Logistics Battalion in Chelyabinsk, at 3 a.m. on New Year's morning, a drunken sergeant bullied Sychev from his bed, tied his legs and forced him to squat down, balancing himself on the balls of his feet. The kid was forced to stay there, squatting for three and a half hours. The pain of it was punctuated by occasional hefty kicks to his ankles. The agony was so pure he thought he would die and that he would be glad to do so. Due to the holidays, it was a couple of days before Private Andrei Sychev got to see a medic at the clinic on the base. His leg was swollen with what looked like blood clots. He was moved swiftly to hospital in Chelyabinsk. There, the news was bad. Gangrene, it seemed, was galloping through his system. The surgeon cut one leg off and rang Andrei's family in Yekaterinburg. He was going to continue sawing but they should come quickly. Their son almost certainly wouldn't survive. The boy lost both legs and his genitals and the tip of his right ring finger before the saw was sheathed. Inconveniently, Private Andrei Sychev didn't die. His mother, Galina, could not be made to shut up about it. An official got in touch with her several times. If she stopped her whining he could offer her an apartment and $100,000. Wouldn't that be nice? Just stop complaining about what you think happened to your son and these keys and this cash are yours. Don't be a martyr. Take it. She kept talking. The great journalist Anna Politkovskaya reported the bribe attempt in *Novaya Gazeta*. It was becoming a big scandal, getting out of hand. In the end they had to hold a trial in Chelyabinsk. At

first it looked like it would be the same old story: in Russia the less you know the better you sleep. A witness who had testified against the sergeant had a sudden change of heart and stopped showing up in court. Others reversed and edited the statements they had originally given to investigators; on mature recollection, they were mistaken. An army general ordered three soldiers not to testify at the trial. They ignored him and testified anyway and the tide turned. The fury of Russian motherhood won the day. The main defendant, Sergeant Alexander Sivyakov, was found guilty of 'exceeding authority'. He got four years' imprisonment, less time served. Two more junior co-defendants received suspended sentences of eighteen months each. Later in 2006, on 7 October – on Vladimir Putin's birthday, as it happened – Anna Politkovskaya, whose words had reddened Kremlin cheeks so many times, was shot dead in the lift of her apartment in Moscow. A Makarov pistol lay discarded at her feet when she was found. The Makarov was for decades the standard military and police side arm in Russia.

Chapter 10

1 In November 2015 a report of the independent commission of WADA accused Mutko of overseeing a large-scale doping programme within Russian sport. It was alleged that Mutko's ministry had undue influence over Rusada. He was banned for life from attending future Olympic Games, though this ruling was overturned by the Court of Arbitration for Sport on appeal in July 2019. He became Deputy Prime Minister of Russia in 2016. In January 2020 he resigned from his role as Deputy Prime Minister.
2 In January 2015 Valentin Maslakov was asked to step down from his coaching position in the wake of WADA's investigation that found evidence of 'a systematic culture of doping in Russian sport'. Sanctions were only issued in cases where absolute proof existed. Maslakov was not sanctioned by WADA but Richard Pound, chair of the investigation, commented that 'it was beyond belief that he would have been unaware of what was going on and, if he was coaching himself, it was beyond belief that his athletes would not have been part of that system as well.' Following his resignation as head coach in January 2015, Maslakov was replaced by Yuriy Borzakovskiy.

Chapter 11

1 In April 2017 Alexei Melnikov was issued with a lifetime ban for breaches of rules on doping. In March 2018 France issued arrest warrants for both Melnikov and the former head of Russian athletics, Valentin Balakhnichev, as part of an investigation into the cover-up of doping.

Chapter 14

1 Styrkina was coach to Svetlana Masterkova, who won gold in the 800 metres and 1500 metres at the Atlanta Olympics. Masterkova never tested positive throughout her career. In 2012 Klyuka received a two-year ban for an 'abnormal index in her biometric passport'. Her ban, along with others handed out at the same time, marked the first time Russia itself had banned its own athletes due to passport abnormalities. The bans came shortly before the 2012 London Olympics and have been viewed as an attempt by Russian authorities to reassure the world that the state was tough on doping.
2 In March 2017 Dr Sergei Portugalov received a lifetime ban from athletics after the Court of Arbitration for Sport said that 'clear evidence' showed him to have doped athletes. The 2015 WADA report had concluded that Portugalov was 'very active in the conspiracy to cover up athletes' positive tests in exchange for a percentage of their winnings'. The report said that over 1000 Russian sports people had benefited from state-sponsored doping.

Chapter 18

1 In 2017 Mariya Savinova received a four-year ban for doping offences and had three years' worth of her results nullified, including her times in Daegu and her gold medal at the 2012 Olympics. She had previously admitted in the course of a 2014 German television documentary to having used oxandrolone, an anabolic steroid. As a consequence of Savinova's forfeiture of the Olympic gold medal, her compatriot Ekaterina Poistogova had her bronze medal upgraded to a silver. Poistogova later received a two-year doping ban.
2 Svetlana Klyuka later received a two-year ban for biological passport abnormalities. The ban was imposed from February 2011 to 2013, and her performances dating back to 2009 were nullified.
3 Yekaterina Kostetskaya was sanctioned for biological passport abnormalities in July 2014. She received a two-year ban and her 2011 and 2012 times were nullified.
4 In 2018 former WADA director David Howman said that a train transporting pre-Olympic Games samples from Russia to a laboratory in Beijing had been intercepted by the FSB (the body that replaced the KGB in post-Soviet Russia) and the samples seemed to have disappeared. The samples were from four race-walkers including Borchin and Olga Kaniskina, both of whom won gold medals at Beijing. These events were highlighted in an affidavit by Dr Grigori Rodchenkov, who also said that the interception had been requested by Chegin. In a discussion that had taken place at the time between WADA and Russian officials, it was claimed Russian law prevented the transportation of bodily samples beyond the state. In June 2016 WADA had discovered that all samples scheduled to leave the state had for many years first been re-routed to Moscow.

5 Borchin won gold in Beijing. At the 2012 London Olympics he collapsed within 2km of the finish line in the 20km event. In 2015 he was given an eight-year ban from the sport retrospective to October 2012 and many of his results were annulled, including all those from August 2009 to October 2012. Kaniskina and Kanaykin were also among a group of walkers who received bans at that time on the basis of the haematological profiles of samples taken under the biological passport programme.

6 Some years later Rodchenkov would state that in 2011 he had been placed under investigation for the trafficking of performance-enhancing drugs to supply Russian athletes and for extorting them for payment to conceal drug tests. Given that this activity was hardly secret, the investigation was considered to be politically motivated. Rodchenkov's suicide attempt led to him being admitted to psychiatric care for two months, by which time the trouble seemed to have passed. He returned to his job and later insisted that the price he had paid to avoid prosecution was his compliance in the grand scheme to provide expert doping support to Russian athletes at Sochi. When the story became public in 2016 the IOC said it had no prior knowledge of the colourful history of the man who oversaw the anti-doping charade at the Sochi Olympics. Interviewed by WADA in 2016, Rodchenkov confirmed that he had destroyed 1,417 samples from Russian athletes in order to hamper WADA's audit of the Moscow laboratory.

7 In an interview with the *Guardian*, Meadows spoke about Yuliya and that meeting. 'For some reason I have always felt she was different. When we raced she would always smile and be friendly. But in Daegu [for the 2011 World Championships] I noticed a very different look on her face when she beat me into third. We were going back into the village, she was really remorseful and told me, "I am really sorry you didn't make the final." There was something behind those eyes. I don't forgive any other Russians but I do forgive her.'

Chapter 19

1 The Sochi Winter Olympics would transpire to be the high-water mark of the Russian dysfunctional sports culture. In 2016 Rodchenkov, who had fled to the US, told the *New York Times* that anti-doping officials, agents of the FSB intelligence agency and Russian coaches and athletes had conspired to cheat on an industrial scale. The FSB, he claimed, tampered with over a hundred samples as part of the operation. He alleged the existence of a so-called Sochi Duchess List that contained the names of thirty-seven Russian athletes whose samples were as a matter of course to be swapped for clean urine samples that they had previously supplied and which had been stored in the FSB command centre in Sochi. This allowed the listed athletes to compete while fully doped. Much of the information that led to the full disclosure of what happened in Sochi flowed from fifteen hours of conversation between Rodchenkov and Vitaly.

2   Russia won eighty-two medals at the 2012 Olympics. Twenty-four gold, twenty-seven silver and thirty-one bronze. Subsequently Russia was stripped of fifteen of those medals, including five golds. A WADA report described Russia as having 'sabotaged' the Games. Lifetime and long-term suspensions were given to ten coaches and athletes. Yuliya's 800 metres rival, Mariya Savinova, who won gold, was among them. A later report, issued after an investigation commissioned by WADA and carried out by Richard McLaren, concluded that Russia had operated 'a state-directed failsafe system' using a 'disappearing positive (test) methodology' from at least late 2011 through August 2015.

Chapter 20

1   In November 2016 an examination of Martynova's (by then using her married surname, Sharmina) biological passport indicated blood doping. The Court of Arbitration for Sport voided the athlete's results from June 2011 to August 2115 and issued a ban from competition for three years backdated to December 2015.

2   In July 2014 Kostetskaya was sanctioned for doping. She received a two-year ban backdated to end in January 2015.

3   In 2017, five years after the race itself, the IOC reassigned the gold medal to Maryam Yusuf Jamal of Bahrain. Pending the outcome of investigations into other finishers, the silver- and bronze-medal positions were left vacant until 2018, when Tomashova was awarded the silver despite herself having served a two-year ban from 2008 to 2010 for manipulating doping samples. Abeba Aregawi of Ethiopia (later Sweden), who finished fifth originally, was given the bronze. She was reported to have failed a drug test in Addis Ababa in January 2016, and voluntarily agreed to a suspension but was reinstated later that year, just before the Rio Olympics, due to insufficient evidence on how long the drug meldonium takes to leave the body. The drug in question had just been banned, in January 2016.

4   Arzhakova was banned for two years from 29 January 2013 for showing an abnormal haemoglobin profile in her biological passport. Her results from 12 July 2011 onwards were nullified.

5   'As well as the doping charges, Russian trio Yulamanova, Zinurova and Klyuka were also suspended for "abnormal indexes in their biometric passports", the first time Russian athletes have been banned for such offences. Yulamanova, 31, finished second in the marathon at the 2010 European Championships in Barcelona. But she was awarded the gold medal after the original winner, Lithuania's Zivile Balciunaite, was disqualified and banned for using steroids. Yulamanova also finished eighth in the marathon at the 2009 World Championships in Berlin. Both Yulamanova's and Klyuka's suspensions have been backdated from February 2012, while 800m indoor European champion Zinurova's ban began in September 2011. Their suspensions mean all three are ineligible to compete at this week's

Russian championships in Cheboksary, and therefore cannot compete at London 2012. "This is the first time athletes have been suspended in Russia because of abnormality of their biometric passports," said Russian Athletics Federation president Valentin Balakhnichev. "We know such practice has been widely used in cycling but unfortunately it's now been the case with our athletes as well. It's a huge loss for our team but their guilt has been proven beyond doubt."' (www.bbc.com/sport/olympics/18697282)

6 In 2013 Marguet's result was again reclassified to take into account Yuliya's ban. Marguet was now upgraded to the silver-medal position, the greatest achievement of her career.

7 While serving an unofficial ban, Alminova decided to train with Nike's controversial Alberto Salazar elite group.

8 Kazarin eventually received a lifetime ban from sport in 2017, having been found guilty of possessing, trafficking and administering banned substances. In 2019 he admitted to having continued working with athletes after his ban. Having grown a beard in an attempt to disguise himself, he was spotted by a drug tester working with athletes at a training camp in Kyrgyzstan. In an interview in 2019, Kazarin said that he had only given drugs to Yuliya 'just so she would go away' as she had been nagging him. He said, when the bans were handed out, that the Russian authorities had treated him and other coaches 'like trash'. For working with Kazarin while he was a banned coach, the Russian 400 metres runner Artyom Denmukhametov received a provisional suspension in 2019. At the same time, it was reported in Russia that banned figures such as Mokhnev and Valery Volkov were also coaching athletes in Russia, while Portugalov was reported to be providing medical advice on nutrition and training through lectures at a Moscow gym.

Chapter 25

1 In November 2015 long-standing IAAF president Lamine Diack and his legal adviser, Habib Cissé, were charged with corruption, money-laundering and conspiracy, having been arrested in Monaco. After two days of questioning by French prosecutors, they were released on bail and officially placed under investigation. In September 2019 the Ethics Board of the IAAF banned Cissé for life and fined him $25,000. They had found him guilty of helping to cover up the doping violations of Russian marathoner Liliya Shobukhova 'and other Russian athletes'. Shobukhova was found to have paid $450,000 in exchange for having her blood passport case slowed down in order to compete at the 2012 Olympic Games. The investigation into the Shobukhova case led to Melnikov and Valentin Balakhnichev, a former IAAF treasurer, being banned for life from athletics for causing 'unprecedented damage'. In January 2020 Cissé began a trial in France on charges of corruption and money-laundering. Melnikov, Balakhnichev and former IAAF president Lamine Diack, former IAAF marketing consultant

Papa Massata Diack and former IAAF anti-doping chief Gabriel Dollé also faced trial. International warrants for Melnikov and Balakhnichev were issued in January 2019 but they remained in Russia as the trial began. They both denied the charges.

2   The foot-dragging of the IAAF in the matter of the Russian doping scandal had been a depressing sideshow all along. The reasons for the IAAF's tardiness would become clear years later, when the January 2020 trial of leading IAAF figures in Paris heard that they had 'established a veritable organised criminal organisation of formidable efficiency, specialising in corruption, money laundering and embezzlement'. By that time, these words would come as no surprise to observers. After the WADA Independent Commission report was delivered in late 2015, Sebastian Coe, the IAAF's new president, had announced that 'This has been a shameful wake-up call.' The alarm had been ringing for quite some time, however, while Coe and his colleagues buried their heads under well-fluffed pillows. When the biological passport system was launched in 2009, the results soon revealed that Russia was operating a massive kamikaze-style system of doping. 'Not only are these athletes cheating their fellow competitors but at these levels are putting their health and even their own lives in very serious danger,' Pierre Weiss, the IAAF general secretary from 2006–11, wrote in a letter dated 14 October 2009 to Valentin Balakhnichev, the Russian athletics president who would later incur a lifetime ban from the sport. Weiss noted that the Russians had already 'recorded some of the highest values ever seen since the IAAF started testing'. He said that tests at the 2009 World Championships in Berlin 'strongly suggest a systematic abuse of blood doping or EPO-related products'. The Russians had won thirteen medals at those championships. After the 2009 Worlds, Weiss told Balakhnichev that no less than Russians, 'including two gold medallists', would have been forced to sit out the competition if the IAAF had enforced the same rules as for some other sports. Before the London Olympics, IAAF internal documents further revealed that the organisation had proposed concealing the doping sanctions of lesser-known Russian athletes. The elite, better-known athletes could not be discreetly made to vanish. On 28 September 2012, after the London Games, another internal brief – this time to the then-IAAF president Lamine Diack – suggested that 42 per cent of tested Russian elite athletes had been dopers. By 2011, the IAAF's new testing regime was flagging so many suspected Russian dopers that officials explored breaking their own rules and those of WADA by dealing with some cases privately, two notes show. An internal IAAF document from 2011 would reveal that the IAAF found it unavoidable to sanction elite Russian athletes who were likely to win medals in London, but suggested 'rapid and discreet' handling for lesser-known Russian athletes. For athletes who agreed to this form of extraordinary rendition removing them from the scene, the IAAF would 'undertake not to publish the sanction'. The suspension itself would be shortened to two years from four, according to a brief dated 5 December 2011 that was sent by IAAF anti-doping director Gabriel Dollé to Diack's legal counsel, Habib Cissé. The

farce that the Russian presence made of several events at the London Games, and their perversion of the entire system in Sochi two years later, had been the inevitable result of wake-up calls that had come years earlier. Buried deep in the WADA report of November 2015 would be a curious paragraph concerning the IAAF: 'Interestingly, however, in September of 2014, the Russian Ministry of Sport requested a meeting with WADA in Lausanne to report that abnormal ABP cases were not dealt with in a timely manner and claimed that ARAF and the Russian athletes had been "blackmailed" by senior IAAF officials to allow athletes with abnormal ABPs to compete in exchange for money. No details were provided at the time, nor since, regarding the identities of the IAAF officials alleged to have been engaged in such blackmail, and no details of any monetary payments have been provided by the Russian Ministry of Sport. The IC is, on the basis of lack of evidence, unable to reach any conclusion in relation to such allegations.'

3 Robertson subsequently requested a drug analysis examination of the tablets at the WADA accredited, anti-doping laboratory at Salt Lake City in the US. The laboratory determined that the tablets contained oxandrolone, dehydrochloromethyltestosterone, mestanolone and methenolone acetate. Each of which is classified as a prohibited item under Code S1, Anabolic Agents.

Chapter 27

1 As well as Russian investigative journalist Anna Politkovskaya, dozens of other Russian journalists have been murdered since 1992 – many shot but a surprising number of them appearing to have accidentally fallen from high windows or balconies.

Chapter 28

1 A Schengen visa, named after the town in Luxembourg where the visa scheme was agreed and established in 1985, is the document issued by the appropriate authorities to the interested party for visiting/travelling to and within the Schengen Area. The Schengen Area comprises twenty-six countries that have agreed to allow free movement of their citizens within this area as a single country. Of the twenty-six countries bound by the Schengen agreement, twenty-two are part of the EU and the other four are part of the EFTA (European Free Trade Area). The Schengen Area covers the majority of European countries, with the most significant exception being the UK.

Chapter 30

1 The curious thing about the story of Bazdyreva was that when Seppelt cut
his original documentary he excised her. She was a nobody. Bazdyreva
had dodged a bullet. The documentary showed footage of her own coach
handing drugs to an athlete so it was possibly unwise therefore for her to turn
up to the Russian National Indoors Championships in February and win the
title out of the blue. She competed at the European Indoor Championships
in Prague in March but was disqualified from her semi-final for stepping
off the track. She won the 800 metres at the Russian Team Championships
in Sochi and went on to win the National title in August in Cheboksary.
WADA investigators had actually approached her in Prague. She had
dismissed them in a squall of righteous indignation. She continued making
herself conspicuous. Before the World Championships in Beijing in August
2015 Seppelt issued a second Russian documentary using the wealth of
material he had. This time Bazdyreva had done enough to earn her moments
of fame. The recording from Lake Issyk-Kul was included. She dropped out
of the World Championship in Beijing at the last minute. Russian Athletics
Federation acting president Vadim Zelichenok said, 'Bazdyreva has decided
not to take part in the World Championships because of the allegations made
in the film . . . we could have included her but she said: "I want to dismiss all
the suspicions surrounding me and carry on training."'

Two weeks before Beijing Vitaly and Yuliya had been brought to the
offices of Carrard & Associés in Lausanne to sign statements testifying to
the authenticity of their recordings. They were informed by lawyers that
several of the athletes concerned would be suspended the day before World
Championships began. They learned later that the athletes were actually
suspended but the sanctions were never publicly announced. The IAAF was
reluctant to have doping as the opening theme in their latest big show.

The always interesting website of the Sports Integrity Initiative ran a short
but fascinating piece after the 2015 Russian National Championships. It
seemed that Seppelt's documentary and the WADA investigation were having
an inhibiting effect on Russian athletes where decades of sanctions had
failed. For a nation preparing for the imminent World Championships, times
were slower right across the board in Cheboksary as Russian athletes tried
not to draw attention to themselves. Bazdyreva benefited from the general
go-slow. 'The 2015 women's 800m winner, Anastasiya Bazdyreva, recorded
the slowest time over the last ten years at the Russian Championships. With
a time of a second over two minutes, she was almost six seconds slower than
2008's winner, Yelena Soboleva.' (http://www.sportsintegrityinitiative.com/
why-are-the-russians-getting-slower/)

In December 2016 the Court of Arbitration for Sport issued decisions on
the cases of both Bazdyreva and Mokhnev. Bazdyreva was found to have
violated IAAF codes on use of prohibited substances and incurred a two-
year period of ineligibility backdated from 24 August 2015. Her results from
April 2014 to August 2015 were erased. Mokhnev was cited as the coach of

Stepanova, Kupina and others. He was found to have violated codes relating to possession, trafficking and administration of banned substances. He received a ten-year ban from December 2016. Bazdyreva didn't go gently and became a favourite of Russian publications for her denunciations of WADA and their 'pseudo investigations'. She was quoted at one stage claiming that WADA officials had held her against her will in Prague: 'So three young meatheads without explaining their reasons try to force a girl into some room in one of the European capitals and I'm being aggressive? I was just scared at that moment.' (RT Online, 27 January 2017)

Chapter 32

1 In an interview with the *New York Times* on 12 May 2016 Dr Grigory Rodchenkov, the director of the Moscow anti-doping laboratory and the scientist in charge of the anti-doping laboratory at the Sochi Winter Olympics, would shed more light on the alcohol story. Rodchenkov said he had developed a cocktail of three anabolic steroids: methenolone, trenbolone and oxandrolone. '"The drugs," Dr. Rodchenkov said, "helped athletes recover quickly after gruelling training regimens, allowing them to compete in top form over successive days . . ." To speed up absorption of the steroids and shorten the detection window, he dissolved the drugs in alcohol — Chivas whiskey for men, Martini vermouth for women . . . Dr. Rodchenkov's formula was precise: one milligram of the steroid mixture for every milliliter of alcohol. The athletes were instructed to swish the liquid around in their mouths, under the tongue, to absorb the drugs.'

Index

365

micro-dosing 293
Ministry for Sport, Russian viii, 178,
  341, 336–7, 341; 'away tests' and
  132; Mutko and *see* Mutko, Vitaly;
  Rusada testing, influence over
  79, 99–100, 109, 110, 114, 129,
  189, 333; Sinev conflict with 99,
  341; Sochi Games and 150–51;
  untouchable athletes, list of 85–6;
  WADA and 114, 336
Mitkov, Andrei 317
Mokhnev, Vladimir 196, 259, 338;
  Portugalov and 109, 123–4; VS
  and 144, 165; YS doping and 64,
  106–8, 113, 118, 119, 120, 121,
  122, 123–4, 252, 291; YS drops as
  coach 166, 251–2; YS first meets
  63; YS IDTM test and 155; YS
  injury before Olympics (2012) and
  165, 251; YS recordings of 251–2,
  254–6; YS sexual relationship with
  28, 29, 106, 120, 165, 185, 186,
  194, 252, 312; YS tuberculosis and
  61, 117, 283
Moscow Anti-Doping Laboratory 18,
  20, 79, 86, 109, 113, 120, 147, 318
Moscow Laboratory, second/secret
  (Laboratory of the Moscow
  Committee of Sport) 126–7, 136,
  342
Moser, Jean-Pierre 41
Mutko, Vitaly 75, 100, 315, 316, 317,
  318, 335, 343, 344

New York, US 7–11, 12, 169–70, 227,
  309
Niggli, Olivier 135, 152
Nike 125, 257, 258, 259
9/11 7–11, 12, 101, 224–5
Nizhny Tagil Athletics club 260–61
Nochevnyy, Sergey 15, 283
'no notice' test 103, 155, 171

Olympics 7; (2000) 52, 159, 324; (2004)
  52, 77; (2008) 20, 21, 43–4, 50,
  54–5, 72, 74, 80, 126, 140–42, 158,
  161, 173, 317; (2010) (Winter) 72,
  73–80, 81, 82, 85, 88, 102, 140,
  150, 341; (2012) 125, 134, 139, 146,
  154, 159, 160, 162, 163, 165, 166,

  168, 170, 172–4, 175, 176, 177, 189,
  238, 239, 255, 263, 267, 314, 341–2;
  (2014) (Winter) 148–51, 229, 247,
  314, 341, 342; (2016) 175, 260, 298,
  314, 323; (2020) 314
out-of-competition doping control 19,
  103, 164
oxandrolone 124, 131, 263, 269, 271, 291

Painter, Trevor 145–6
Pecherina, Yevgeniya 315
peptides 144
Pervakov, Sergey 76, 82, 84, 85–7
Physical Culture and Sports Committee
  of Kursk region 177
Pioline, Denis 158
Pleskach-Styrkina, Svetlana 172
Poistogova, Ekaterina 173, 263
Portugalov, Sergei 167, 210, 259; athlete
  biological passport (ABP) and 134,
  179, 180, 181, 196; away tests,
  protocol for 132; client/supplier
  conditions with YS established
  122; end preparation of athletes,
  expresses wish to 181, 351; 'first
  class plus' category of athletes
  144–5, 146–7, 164, 241, 293, 294;
  Kazarin and 168, 175, 176, 181,
  270; Olympics (2012), prediction
  of YS performance at 127, 139;
  relevance of doping test results, on
  115; Savinova and 144–5, 164, 166,
  241, 294; VS and 163, 176, 196,
  296, 297–8; WADA and 136; YS
  athlete biological passport (ABP)
  and 134, 196; YS doping overseen
  by 120, 121, 122, 123–4, 125, 126,
  127, 128, 130, 131, 132, 134, 136,
  138, 139, 144–5, 146–7, 154–5,
  161–2, 163, 164, 166, 167, 179, 180,
  181, 194, 210, 217, 220, 296–301,
  339; YS, ends working relationship
  with 161–2, 296; YS first meets
  109–10; YS, shift in attitude
  towards 154–5, 161–2, 163–4, 296;
  YS recordings of 219, 296–301,
  305; YS texts sample numbers to
  124, 132, 147, 161
Pound, Dick 315, 316, 317, 318
Pravda 32, 321

Stepanov, Vitaly – *continued*
personnel, meets in Boston (2011)
134–5, 220; WADA, VS first
outlines Russian doping culture
to members of, Vancouver Winter
Olympics 74, 75–80; wedding
66–70, 82; whistle-blower status
217–18, 236, 314, 318, 322; YS,
approach towards doping of in
WADA correspondence 112–13,
120, 121, 130, 135, 139–40, 142–3,
151, 152–8, 160–61, 169, 171, 181,
186, 201, 215, 228, 229, 327–52;
YS attempts to leave 88–96; YS,
considers divorcing 72–3, 88–92,
93–7, 102, 111, 128, 138, 183–4,
185–203, 206, 209–11, 215,
222, 281, 298; YS, dates 23–9;
YS family and 57, 58, 66–70,
72; YS, first meets viii, 3–15;
YS, pacemaker for 159–61; YS,
proposes marriage to 57–8
Stepanov (née Rusanova), Yuliya:
amateur races 62, 63–4; AndroGel
(testosterone gel), use of 144–5;
athlete biological passport (ABP)
system and 133–4, 155, 168,
173–4, 179–81, 194–6, 206, 219,
300–301, 350–51; athletics career
(races/championships) *see individual
championship and race name*; Berlin,
exile/life in vii, viii, 303–6,
308–11; Berlin, Seppelt first hosts
VS and in 249–51; boyfriend
(Vladimir) 185–6, 197, 200–201,
210–11; child *see* Stepanov,
Robert; childhood 11–12, 25–8,
34–9, 58–65, 72, 82, 91–2, 283;
coaches *see* Kazarin, Vladimir *and*
Mokhnev, Vladimir; 'corridor'
(parameters within which athletes'
ABP blood levels are tested) and
269–70; doping, begins 63–4,
118–19; DW meets vii, viii; EPO
doping 106–9, 113, 119–20, 121,
123, 131–2, 133, 134, 141, 154, 155,
209, 269, 329–31; EPO positive
test sample, pays bribe to cover
up 106–9; family *see individual
family member name*; 'first class plus'

category of athletes and 144–7, 164,
241, 293, 294; flees Russia 301–2;
frozen urine, instructed to keep
clean for unforeseen situations 124;
Germany, leaves 321; honeymoon
70, 72; human growth hormone
doping 121, 181, 269, 291–2, 329;
IDTM test on, WADA orders
155–8, 171; Kazarin and *see*
Kazarin, Vladimir; Kemp offers to
meet 171; Kurchatov lady forsees
fortune of 284–6; Kursk payment
of performance monies to 176–9,
216; Lake Issyk-Kul training camp,
Kyrgyzstan 138, 165, 265–81,
288, 290, 298; life threatened in
Germany 310–11; Meadows, guilty
talk with in Daegu 145–6; medal,
first international 134; Melnikov
and *see* Melnikov, Alexei; Mokhnev
and *see* Mokhnev, Vladimir;
motivation for revealing Russian
doping culture vii–viii; name
change 223; Olympics (2012),
injury rules out participation in
165–6, 167, 171, 172, 175, 182, 201,
251, 255, 286; Olympics (2016) and
323; Oral Turinabol doping 119;
out-of-competition Rusada test
164; oxandrolone doping 124, 131,
269, 271, 291; Parabolan doping
124; personal best times, effects
of doping on 118–20, 125, 127,
139, 298; police, Moscow, runs for
13–14, 24–5, 219, 223, 309–10;
Portugal training camps 131, 138,
162–4; Portugalov oversees doping
regimen of *see* Portugalov, Sergei;
pragmatist viii, 64; prize money
83, 96, 164; races/championships
*see individual championship and
race name*; recordings/tapings of
colleagues *see individual colleague
name*; Robertson meeting in
Istanbul and 219–21; Rusada,
informs VS of the true purpose
of 4, 84; running, first discovers
37, 38–9, 62; Russian National
team, becomes member of 120;
Savinova and *see* Savinova, Mariya;

senate hearing in Washington,
speaks at 322; testosterone and 118,
121, 123, 131, 132, 144, 154, 181,
269, 323, 329, 339; texts sample
numbers to Portugalov 132, 147,
161; *Top Secret Doping – How Russia
Makes Its Winners* (documentary)
and 253, 304, 306, 309–11 *see also*
recordings/tapings of colleagues;
Trental, injects 123; tuberculosis
24, 61, 117–18, 283; two-year
ban from athletics 190, 194 5,
200–208, 210, 216, 218, 239, 257,
260, 261, 262, 268, 276, 290, 301,
307; United States, life/exile in
viii, 224–5, 321–6; United States,
visits with VS 169–72; VS, attempts
to leave 88–96, 185–203, 185–203,
206, 209–11, 215, 222; VS, cheats
on 185–7; VS, considers divorcing
72–3, 88–92, 93–7, 102, 183–4,
185–203, 206, 209–11, 215, 222,
281, 298; VS, dates 3–15, 23–9;
VS and family of 57, 58, 66–70,
72; VS, first meets viii, 3–15; VS
marriage proposal 57–8; VS as
pacemaker for 159–61; VS WADA
correspondence and 112–13, 120,
121, 130, 135, 139–40, 142–3,
151, 152–8, 160–61, 169, 171, 181,
186, 201, 215, 228, 229, 327–52;
WADA knowledge of doping
79–80, 111, 112–13, 120, 121,
130, 135, 136, 139–40, 142–3,
151, 152–8, 160–61, 169, 171, 181,
186, 201, 210, 215, 217–18, 220,
228, 229, 232, 235–6, 306–8,
311, 327–52; WADA, statement/
letter to outlining Russian doping
system 217–18, 220, 232, 235–6;
wedding 66–70, 82; whistle-blower
status 217–18, 236, 314, 318; White
House, invitation to 322–3
Styrkina, Svetlana 105, 330
Sunday Times 232, 318–20

testosterone 118, 121, 123, 131, 132,
144, 154, 181, 269, 323, 329, 339
Tomashova, Tatyana 173
Top Secret Doping – How Russia Makes

Its Winners (documentary): editing
263–5; filming/interviews of VS
and YS 253; German television
broadcast 304; opening credits
vii–viii; origins of 233–4, 235–8,
244, 246–8, 249–51; reaction to
broadcast 304–5, 309–26; release
date 253–4, 273, 297 *see also*
Seppelt, Hajo
Trofimov, Yevgeny 317
Tutova, Russia 26–7, 28, 59–60
Tygart, Travis 321
Tyutchev, Fyodor 1

United States Anti-Doping Agency 316,
321
Untouchables, The (film) 17
Ural Great basketball club 31, 33

Vaganova, Natalia 82, 86
Vatutin, Andrey 31, 33
Venofer 131
Verbitskaya, Irina 45–6
Vessey, Maggie 145
Virupaev, Konstantin 100, 114, 332,
335, 336
VNIIFK Institute (All Russian Research
Institute of Physical Culture and
Sport) 297–301

World Anti-Doping Agency (WADA)
19, 33, 41, 42, 100, 229; Beijing
Olympic Games Outreach
programme 43–4, 55, 72, 74, 80,
140–42, 158; Code *see* World Anti-
Doping Code; dirty samples sent to
national anti-doping organisations
86; IDTM and 151–8, 171, 306–8;
independent commission (IC)/
Pound report 315, 316, 317; lifetime
bans for doping, recommends five
Russian runners receive (2015) 173;
McLaren Report and 316; national
doping control, systems, inability
to investigate 79, 136–7, 140,
253–4; out-of-competition doping
control 19, 103, 164; Reedie and
315, 316, 317; Robertson and *see*
Robertson, Jack; Rodchenkov
arrest and 143; Rusada, reliance